INTELLIGENT ANALYSIS OF
FUNDUS IMAGES
Methods and Applications

Series On Deep Learning Neural Networks

Series Editors: Daniel Graupe *(The Univ Of Illinois At Chicago, USA)* &
Derong Liu *(Univ Of Illinois At Chicago, USA)*

Published

Vol. 1   *Intelligent Analysis of Fundus Images: Methods and Applications*
by Yuanyuan Chen, Yi Zhang & Jie Zhong

Series on Deep Learning Neural Networks – Volume 1

INTELLIGENT ANALYSIS OF
FUNDUS IMAGES
Methods and Applications

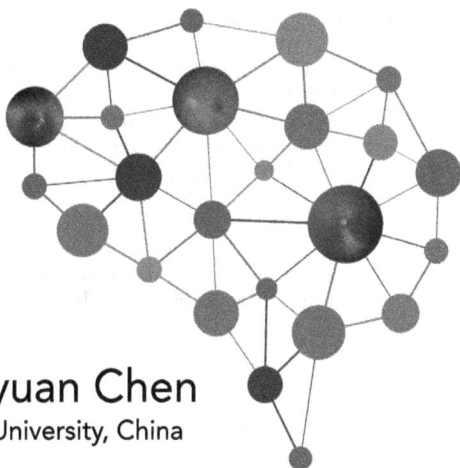

Yuanyuan Chen
Sichuan University, China

Jie Zhong
University of Electronic Science
and Technology of China, China

Zhang Yi
Sichuan University, China

World Scientific

NEW JERSEY · LONDON · SINGAPORE · BEIJING · SHANGHAI · HONG KONG · TAIPEI · CHENNAI · TOKYO

Published by

World Scientific Publishing Co. Pte. Ltd.

5 Toh Tuck Link, Singapore 596224

USA office: 27 Warren Street, Suite 401-402, Hackensack, NJ 07601

UK office: 57 Shelton Street, Covent Garden, London WC2H 9HE

Library of Congress Cataloging-in-Publication Data
Names: Chen, Yuanyuan (Of Sichuan University), author. |
    Zhong, Jie (Ophthalmologist), author. | Yi, Zhang, author.
Title: Intelligent analysis of fundus images : methods and applications /
    Yuanyuan Chen, Sichuan University, China,
    Jie Zhong, University of Electronic Science and Technology of China, China,
    Zhang Yi, Sichuan University, China.
Other titles: Series on deep learning neural networks ; v. 1.
Description: New Jersey : World Scientific, [2023] | Series: Series on deep learning
    neural networks ; vol. 1 | Includes bibliographical references and index.
Identifiers: LCCN 2022058148 | ISBN 9789811270369 (hardcover) |
    ISBN 9789811270376 (ebook for institutions) | ISBN 9789811270383 (ebook for individuals)
Subjects: MESH: Retina--diagnostic imaging | Retinal Diseases--diagnostic imaging |
    Neural Networks, Computer | Deep Learning
Classification: LCC RE551 | NLM WW 270 | DDC 617.7/35075--dc23/eng/20230328
LC record available at https://lccn.loc.gov/2022058148

British Library Cataloguing-in-Publication Data
A catalogue record for this book is available from the British Library.

For any available supplementary material, please visit
https://www.worldscientific.com/worldscibooks/10.1142/13249#t=suppl

Desk Editors: Logeshwaran Arumugam/Steven Patt

Typeset by Stallion Press
Email: enquiries@stallionpress.com

Preface

Visual impairment is one of the major health problems worldwide. Fundus lesions are an important cause of irreversible blindness in patients. Fundus diseases not only seriously threaten people's ocular health and quality of life but also impose a huge burden on the socioeconomy. Early detection of fundopathy prevents approximately 80% of visual disturbances. However, most patients cannot evaluate their own risk because of the unapparent symptoms at the early stage of ophthalmopathy. Specialized fundus examination and diagnosis are essential to prevent blindness. The huge number of patients with fundus disease is in huge contrast to the resource for diagnosis and treatment of fundus disease which is not fully imbalanced in our country.

With the deep integration of artificial intelligence (AI) and medicine, intelligent medicine has been booming. Many important theoretical achievements and successful applications continue to emerge.

This book is oriented to deep neural network methods for intelligent analysis of fundus imaging. In response to many blinding fundus diseases that people suffer in different periods of time, various image acquisition devices and different fundus image analysis tasks are elaborated. In this book, starting from the actual fundus disease analysis tasks, we introduce different deep neural network models, applied systems, and application results, with the aim of providing theoretical and experimental reference basis for researchers in this direction.

About the Authors

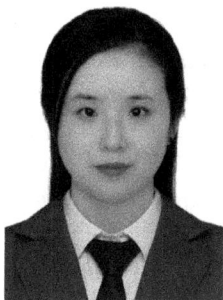

Yuanyuan Chen received her BA in pattern recognition and intelligent systems from Shanghai Jiaotong University in 2007, and then she became a lecturer for teaching and research in the Department of Computer Science at Sichuan University. She received her Ph.D. in machine intelligence from Sichuan University in 2015. Currently, she is an associate professor and master supervisor at Sichuan University.

She is a Director of Sichuan artificial intelligence society. Her research chiefly focuses on artificial intelligence. She has always been dedicated to the research of the theory and applications of neural networks and medical image analysis. She has published more than 30 journal articles in this field.

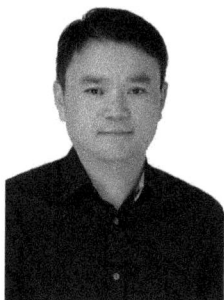

Jie Zhong is a chief physician at Sichuan Provincial People's Hospital. He is currently the Vice Director of Ophthalmology at Sichuan Academy of Medical Sciences Sichuan Provincial People's Hospital. His recent research interests include high myopia fundus disease, retinal detachment, and retinopathy of prematurity.

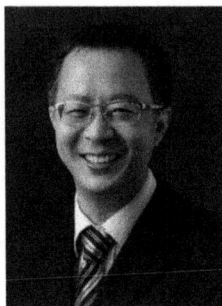

Zhang Yi is the current Director of the Intelligent Interdisciplinary Research Center at Sichuan University. He is a foreign academician of the Russian Academy of Engineering. He received his Ph.D. in mathematics from the Chinese Academy of Sciences in 1994.

He was a Senior Visiting Scholar at the University of Sheffield, UK, from 1989 to 1990; a Research Fellow at the Chinese University of Hong Kong from 1990 to 2001; and a Research Fellow at the National University of Singapore from 2001 to 2002. He served as the Dean of the College of Computer Science, Sichuan University, from 2008 to 2017. In 2019, he won the State Natural Science Award.

He has published more than 300 publications, including being the co-author of three books: *Convergence Analysis of Recurrent Neural Networks* (Kluwer Academic Publisher, 2004), *Neural Networks: Computational Models and Applications* (Springer, 2007), and *Subspace Learning of Neural Networks* (CRC Press, 2010). He was an Associate Editor of *IEEE Transactions on Neural Networks and Learning Systems* (2009–2012). He was promoted to IEEE Fellow in 2016 for Contributions to *Convergence Theory for Neural Networks and Subspace Learning*. Currently, he is an Associate Editor of *IEEE Transactions on Cybernetics* (2014–present).

Acknowledgments

This book has been made possible by the work of many people. I would like to thank and acknowledge Professor Zhang Yi. Professor Zhang Yi started to lead us to the research of intelligent medicine in the summer of 2017. He guided us to integrate AI and Ophthalmology, to delve deeper into neural network models, and to constantly explore applied practices, thus it could yield such fruitful results. My sincere thanks to the collaborating physicians who helped us to collect and label the fundus images. I also want to thank all of the members of DeepEyes group in Machine Intelligence Lab at Sichuan University. They contributed a lot on data collection and preprocessing, model construction and experiments, and the applied systems development.

Contents

Preface   v

About the Authors   vii

Acknowledgments   ix

1. **Introduction**   1
   1.1 Current Status of Fundus Lesions 1
   1.2 The Progress of Artificial Intelligence in Intelligent
       Medical Diagnosis 3
   1.3 DNN and the Diagnosis of Ocular Fundus Lesions . .   6
   1.4 The Main Content of This Book   9

2. **Automated Analysis for Retinopathy of**
   Prematurity by Deep Neural Networks   11
   2.1 Methods 12
       2.1.1 Image labeling 12
       2.1.2 Deep neural networks 14
       2.1.3 Experts' comparisons 16
       2.1.4 Testing of the DeepROP system under
             clinical settings 17
   2.2 Results 19
       2.2.1 Large-scale ROP datasets 19
       2.2.2 Performance of the model 21

      2.2.3 Comparison of the model with human experts   22

      2.2.4 DeepROP website and clinical test 24

  2.3 Discussions 25

3. DeepROP: An Automated ROP Screening System   **27**

  3.1 Retinopathy of Prematurity 28

  3.2 Related Works 32

      3.2.1 Traditional methods for diagnosis of ROP . . . 32

      3.2.2 Deep neural networks for diagnosis of ROP . . 33

  3.3 Data and Methodology 35

      3.3.1 Data 35

      3.3.2 Methodology 39

  3.4 Experimental Setup and Results 42

      3.4.1 Experimental setup 42

      3.4.2 Results 44

  3.5 Clinical Application of DeepROP 51

      3.5.1 System framework 53

      3.5.2 System implementation 55

      3.5.3 Clinical application 60

  3.6 Conclusion 60

4. Diagnosis of Diabetic Retinopathy Using Deep Neural Networks   **63**

  4.1 Introduction 63

  4.2 Related Works 66

      4.2.1 Related dataset 67

      4.2.2 Traditional practice 67

      4.2.3 Deep convolutional neural network approaches 68

  4.3 Overview 69

  4.4 Dataset Construction 71

  4.5 Data Preprocessing and Augmentation 72

      4.5.1 Preprocessing 72

      4.5.2 Augmentation 75

  4.6 Model 76

  4.7 Experiments 79

      4.7.1 Experimental setup 79

      4.7.2 Details of learning 81

      4.7.3 Results 82

      4.7.4 Visualization 82

  4.8 Model Deployment and Clinical Evaluation 84

  4.9 Conclusion 86

5. Automated Identification and Grading System of Diabetic Retinopathy Using Deep Neural Networks   **89**

  5.1 Related Works 90

      5.1.1 Traditional methods for DR diagnosis 90

      5.1.2 Deep learning for DR diagnosis 91

  5.2 Dataset 92

      5.2.1 Materials 92

      5.2.2 Grading standard 93

      5.2.3 Manual grading 95

      5.2.4 Preprocessing of retinal images 96

      5.2.5 Performance comparison 97

      5.2.6 Data augmentation 97

  5.3 Model and Methodology 98

      5.3.1 Aim and objective 98

      5.3.2 Architecture and strategy of ensemble model . 100

      5.3.3 Ensemble strategy 100

      5.3.4 Transfer learning at the first part 101

      5.3.5 Design of customized Standard Deep Neural Network (SDNN) at the second part 101

  5.4 Experiments 103

      5.4.1 Configuration 103

      5.4.2 Strategy 104

      5.4.3 Metrics 107

      5.4.4 Identification system 108

      5.4.5 Grading system 109

      5.4.6 Analysis of experiments 115

  5.5 Discussion 120

  5.6 DeepDR: An AI System for DR Diagnosis 122

  5.7 Conclusion 125

6. Automated Segmentation of Macular Edema in OCT Using Deep Neural Networks   **127**

  6.1 Introduction 128

6.2 Related Works 132
    6.2.1 Traditional methods for segmenting macular
        edema 132
    6.2.2 Deep neural networks for segmenting macular
        edema 133
6.3 Methodology 134
    6.3.1 Atrous spatial pyramid pooling 134
    6.3.2 Stochastic atrous spatial pyramid pooling . . . 137
6.4 Experimental Setup and Results 140
    6.4.1 Experimental setup 140
    6.4.2 Results 143
6.5 DeepOCT: An AI System for Macular Edema Lesion
    Segmentation 152
6.6 Conclusion 154

**7. DeepUWF: An Automated Ultrawide-field
Fundus Screening System via Deep Learning**   **157**

7.1 Introduction 158
7.2 Related Works 159
    7.2.1 Deep learning with traditional imaging
        technology 159
    7.2.2 Deep learning with emerging UWF imaging
        technology 160
7.3 Dataset 160
    7.3.1 Materials 160
    7.3.2 Annotation standard 161
    7.3.3 Annotation result 161
    7.3.4 Preprocessing of UWF images 162
    7.3.5 Data augmentation 166
7.4 Model and Methodology 166
    7.4.1 Aim and objective 166
    7.4.2 Strategy and framework 167
    7.4.3 Selection of feature extractors 167
    7.4.4 Design of customized classifiers 170
    7.4.5 Performance metrics 171
7.5 Experiments 171
    7.5.1 Experimental setup 171
    7.5.2 Screening system 172
    7.5.3 Diagnostic system 175

7.6 Discussion 177
    7.6.1 Image optimization 177
    7.6.2 Medical implication 179
    7.6.3 Limitations 180
    7.6.4 Future work 180
7.7 Conclusion 180

8. **DeepUWF-Plus: Automatic Fundus Identification and Diagnosis System Based on Ultrawide-field Fundus Imaging**   183

8.1 Related Works 184
    8.1.1 Deep learning with traditional imaging technology 184
    8.1.2 Deep learning with emerging UWF imaging technology 184
8.2 Dataset 185
    8.2.1 Materials 185
    8.2.2 Annotation standard 186
    8.2.3 Annotation details 187
    8.2.4 Data preprocessing and augmentation 189
8.3 Model and Methodology 189
    8.3.1 Aim 189
    8.3.2 Feature extractors 191
    8.3.3 Custom classifications 192
    8.3.4 Class imbalance 194
    8.3.5 Evaluation metrics 194
8.4 Experiments 195
    8.4.1 Experimental setup 195
    8.4.2 Experimental design 196
    8.4.3 Screening system 196
    8.4.4 Sign identification system 197
    8.4.5 Disease diagnosis system 199
    8.4.6 Result 200
    8.4.7 Comparative experiments 206
    8.4.8 Generalization performance 207
8.5 Discussion 207
    8.5.1 Comparison of the two strategies 207
    8.5.2 Model performance 209

8.5.3   Medical implication 210

8.5.4   Research limitations 212

8.5.5   Future work 212

8.6   DeepUWF: An AI System for Multiple Fundus
Diseases Diagnosis 213

8.7   Conclusion 214

Bibliography   215

Index   229

Chapter 1

Introduction

1.1 Current Status of Fundus Lesions

Vision health is an important part of physical health. Ophthalmology, its related discipline, studies diseases that occur in the visual system, including the eyeball and its associated tissues. Ophthalmic diseases include blinding eye diseases and non-blinding eye diseases. According to one 2020 ophthalmology industry research report, there are more than 2.2 billion people living with visual impairments worldwide, and more than one billion people suffer from moderate or above visual impairment or blindness due to irreversible diseases. Ocular fundus disease is the first culprit of irreversible blindness; its patients account for 54.7% of all blindness patients, indicating that these diseases seriously threaten people's eye health.

Ocular fundus disease refers to inflammation, tumors of the retina, choroid, optic nerve and vitreous body, various types of vascular disease, various degenerative diseases, and ocular diseases caused by multi-system diseases. It is a common disease type in ophthalmology. Common fundus diseases include age-related macula degeneration (AMD), cataracts, diabetic retinopathy (DR), retinopathy of prematurity (ROP), macular edema (ME), and pathological myopia (PM). In 2020, the total number of myopia patients in China over five years of age exceeded 700 million, and the incidence rate could be estimated at 50.86–51.36%. The number of cataract patients in China increased from 75.2 million in 2002 to 125 million in 2017, a compound growth rate of 3.47%. The *"Big Data Report on Fundus*

Diseases of Chinese People" stated: "The abnormal fundus examination rate of people over 60 years old is higher than 21.39%, that is, one in five people over 60 years old has an abnormal fundus". In addition, according to the *"Report on the Status of Nutrition and Chronic Diseases of Chinese Residents (2020)"*, China is home to 420 million people suffering from hypertension, 200 million people with dyslipidemia, and 121 million people suffering from diabetes, ranking first in the world. Fundus disease is a common complication of a series of chronic diseases. For example, DR is the main cause of blindness in diabetic patients. The *"China Type II Diabetes Prevention Guidelines (2017 Edition)"*, released in January 2018, also pointed out that DR is the first irreversible blindness disease to be prevalent among working-age people and that the prevalence of DR in diabetic patients in China is as high as 24.7–37.5%; in short, three to four million diabetic patients are blinded by DR every year. It can accordingly be observed that the eye health problem in my country is very serious. By 2050, due to the aging of the global population and population growth, the number of people blinded by fundus diseases in China may nearly triple.

Faced with the severe situation of fundus diseases, it is clear that comprehensive fundus screening, early diagnosis, and early treatment are key to preventing patients with fundus diseases from being harmed. The methods currently used for the diagnosis of fundus diseases mainly include ophthalmoscope examination, optical coherence tomography (OCT), fundus angiography, and fundus imaging. Fundus imaging includes fundus color Doppler ultrasound examination and ultrawide-angle fundus imaging examination (UWF).

No matter which method is used, the detection and diagnosis of fundus diseases rely heavily on ophthalmologists and professional fundus readers. However, there are only around 40,000 ophthalmologists in China of which only about 1,000 are engaged in medical services and disease research. Compared with the huge number of fundus disease patients, these figures indicate a serious shortage of ophthalmologists. In addition, there are significant disparities between the levels of medical care available in various regions in China. In summary, the main reasons for the high prevalence of eye diseases in China are the uneven distribution, or sometimes total lack, of various ophthalmic resources. For example, 87% of DR patients in China seek care at medical institutions below the county level, while basic diagnosis and treatment measures and technologies for diabetes are only available at tertiary medical institutions. Data show that 70% of diabetic patients have not received standardized ophthalmological treatment, and about 90% of DR patients with indications for treatment are not treated in time. For ROP, moreover, the research and screening work is uncommon and uneven. Chu and Wang (2012) investigated more than 50 hospitals in 17 regions from 1994 to 2010 and found that the detection rate of the screening was ranged from 2.2% to 48.7%; notably, the detection rate in East China, where ROP screening is conducted earlier and more frequently, was similar at 2.33–48.7%. Moreover, the multi-center investigation of ROP examined 22 units in seven regions from 2010 to 2012 identifying a detection rate of 15.2% (2.8–31.3%) (Zhou *et al.*, 2015). It can accordingly be observed that screening and diagnosis practices for fundus diseases are severely underdeveloped and require significant attention. The training of ophthalmologists and medical personnel is a long-term process, meaning that more training cannot solve the huge problems that exist as soon as required. Due to the huge number of patients with fundus diseases, the lack of adequately trained medical staff, and the labor-intensive nature of fundus screening methods, among other factors, a large number of computer-assisted and automatic fundus imaging screening and diagnosis methods are currently under development.

1.2 The Progress of Artificial Intelligence in Intelligent Medical Diagnosis

Artificial intelligence (AI) is not a recent idea. The concept of AI was first proposed at the Dartmouth Conference of 1956 by John McCarthy, who defined it as "the development of intelligent machines science and technology". Therefore, 1956 has also been referred to as the first year of artificial intelligence. Subsequently, in 1957, Rosenblatt proposed the earliest model of neurons in machine learning artificial neural network theory, known as the perceptron, which gave rise to the first wave of artificial intelligence. In 1967, Cover and Hart proposed the K-nearest neighbor algorithm (Cover and Hart, 1967) based on classification and regression, which enabled a computer to perform simple pattern recognition. In the same year, however, Marvin Minsky outlined the limitations of artificial neural networks in the book Perceptrons. At the same time, with the successive failures in the field of artificial intelligence research, people's optimistic expectations for artificial intelligence have been severely hit, so artificial. The development of intelligence has entered a trough. After several years of precipitation, in 1982, Hopfield proposed a typical full-feedback Hopfield network, which initiated the early research on recurrent neural networks. However, the Hopfield network did not cause a big sensation due to its defect of being easily trapped in a local minimum. Until 1986, under the efforts of Hinton and David E. Rumelhart *et al.*, a backpropagation algorithm suitable for multi-layer perceptrons was proposed to deal with non-uniformity by adding a hidden layer between the input layer and the output layer. Linear problem. The proposal of the BP algorithm set off the second wave of artificial intelligence. Many deep learning network models proposed today use the BP algorithm. In 1998, Hinton's student Yann LeCun and others proposed the first multi-layer convolutional neural network LeNet which achieved good results in handwritten digit recognition. However, due to the limitations of computer capabilities and the "gradient disappearance" of the BP algorithm in multi-layer neural networks, artificial intelligence has entered a bottleneck period.

In 2006, (Hinton and Salakhutdinov, 2006) formally put forward the concept of "deep learning" in a paper published in *Science* magazine. Through unsupervised learning method, layer by layer greedy training provided new ideas for solving the problem of "gradient disappearance". The neural network, known as deep learning, returned to the public eye, but there were still many controversies about deep learning at that time. In 2011, the ReLU activation function was proposed, which further brought hope to solving the "gradient disappearance" problem in deep learning training. In 2012, the AlexNet proposed by Hinton and his student Alex won the championship in the ImageNet competition in one fell swoop (Krizhevsky *et al.*, 2012), with an accuracy rate far surpassing the second place, setting off another climax of deep learning. The reason for AlexNet's dominance is the use of ReLU as the activation function and the use of GPU to greatly reduce the training time. In the following years, a large number of excellent deep neural network models have emerged, such as GoogleNet (Szegedy *et al.*, 2015), VGG (Simonyan and Zisserman, 2014), and ResNet (He *et al.*, 2016b), and artificial intelligence has entered a stage of rapid development. Until 2016, the AlphaGo Go robot developed by Google based on deep learning defeated Li Shishi, a nine-dan Go player. This event marked the beginning of a new era of artificial intelligence. Various terms such as "deep learning", "reinforced learning", and "decision-making network" appeared in various media, forums, columns, etc., and once became a hot topic of discussion in all walks of life. AlphaGo's victory benefited from the powerful "learning" ability of deep learning, by learning the chess-boards that have been played, learning and accumulating experience in continuous contact and actual combat.

In deep learning, by building a multi-layer neural network, extracting features layer by layer, and inputting the results to the next layer, the computer can automatically extract information from massive amounts of data. Deep learning does not require human intervention. It uses rich case data as input data to obtain a pre-diction result, and then adjusts the model parameters by passing the error between the prediction result and the real result between each layer of the model, and continuously loops this. The process stops when the desired effect is achieved. It can be seen that, compared with traditional machine learning methods that are usually composed of multiple independent modules, deep learning is a network that automatically extracts features and strengthens learning and train-ing, and has end-to-end characteristics. Based on these characteris-tics of deep learning and the feat of the intelligent Go robot AlphaGo defeating human professional Go players, it brings new hopes to the further development of deep learning and lays the foundation for the industrialization of deep learning in various fields, such as medical treatment and transportation, finance, and other fields. Nowadays, scientific and technological research in the field of artificial intelli-gence has become a global scientific research hotspot. Among them, the breakthrough progress and achievements in the field of computer vision have brought hope to the application of artificial intelligence in various fields and aroused the interest of more industries. And smart medicine is also the field with the largest development space and the easiest to break through.

In 2018, Abelson *et al.* (2018) published in *Science* a machine learning method that is expected to be able to predict leukemia five years in advance. In August of the same year, the U.S. Food and Drug Administration FDA approved for the first time a product developed using deep learning technology: an AI-based workflow optimization combination product to assist radiologists in triage work. At the same time, the Google DeepMind team also published an intelligent system in *Nature Medicine* that identifies nearly 50 eye diseases based on optical coherence tomography (OCT) data (De Fauw *et al.*, 2018). In 2020, Zhongshan Ophthalmology Center published the world's first artificial intelligence-based ophthalmic disease screening guidance system based on nearly 100,000 ultrawide-area fundus color photos on *Science* (Li *et al.*, 2020). Deep learning technology has made small achievements in the medical field, especially its powerful "feature learning" ability has been fully utilized in medical imaging. Nevertheless, in the face of the diversity of medical cases and the complex environment of clinical applications, intelligent medical research has a long way to go.

1.3   DNN and the Diagnosis of Ocular Fundus Lesions

Clinically, ophthalmologists can directly observe the fundus of the patient through ophthalmoscopes or diagnose a large number of fundus diseases based on auxiliary materials such as color Doppler ultrasound images of the patient's fundus. The fundus color Doppler ultrasound photos allow doctors to see clearly the tissue structure of the fundus and analyze whether there are abnormalities, that is, to detect lesions based on the images, and then propose treatment plans based on detailed screening and diagnosis results. Therefore, the analysis of fundus images includes lesion detection, fundus disease screening, and diagnostic grading which are the first steps in the treatment of fundus diseases. Using fundus images to segment lesions and important biomarkers of fundus diseases, diagnosis and grading, etc., corresponds exactly to tasks such as segmentation, detection, and classification in deep learning. Therefore, the application of deep learning technology in the computer field to fundus imaging as an auxiliary means for ophthalmologists to diagnose and treat fundus diseases is determined by its clinical characteristics. The use of artificial intelligence technology to solve clinical problems is also an inevitable choice for the development of the times.

In recent years, in the scientific clinical research of ophthalmology, AI fundus imaging has received close and extensive attention, and various deep learning-based fundus screening software has quickly landed, a series of automatic diagnosis and screening methods based on deep learning, and lesion segmentation networks have been proposed. The United States, the United Kingdom, and other countries have long carried out AI medical research that combines the field of ophthalmology with the field of artificial intelligence. A large number of research results show that artificial intelligence, especially deep learning technology, is used in fundus diseases, such as diabetic retinopathy and retinopathy of prematurity. Glaucoma, cataract, and other ocular fundus diseases have significant effects in the detection and diagnosis of grading. In 2016, Google researchers and American and Indian doctors established a fundus dataset of nearly 130,000 fundus color ultrasound photos, and each image recorded the evaluation results of 3–7 ophthalmologists. At the same time, Google's DeepMind team published on *JAMA* the first use of GoogLeNet deep neural network to develop an artificial intelligence system for detecting diabetic retinopathy, which has attracted widespread attention in the industry. In the same year, Daniel E. Worrall *et al.* (2016) used GoogLeNet's pretraining model to achieve the diagnostic classification of ROP additional diseases. This is the first attempt to apply deep learning technology to the diagnostic classification of neonatal retinopathy. In February 2018, *cell* published a breakthrough achievement in artificial intelligence and ophthalmology as its cover article. The research is based on a deep learning system for diagnosis and treatment of two types of blinding fundus diseases: macular degeneration and diabetic macular edema. Through diagnosis and corresponding referral and treatment recommendations, the system has achieved an accuracy of more than 95% in clinical trials. This breakthrough has made the intelligent medical business, especially AI fundus imaging, a big step forward. In September of the same year, the first phase of the research results were published in the top medical journal *Nature Medicine*. In January 2020, Zhongshan Eye Center developed the world's first artificial fundus screening guidance system based on nearly 100,000 ultrawide-angle fundus color ultrasound images (Li *et al.*, 2020). In August of the same year, the National

Medical Products Administration (NMPA) certified two screening softwares for diabetic retinopathy. This is also the first batch of artificial intelligence-based ophthalmic diagnosis and treatment assistance systems that have obtained NMPA certification in China. In July 2021, the Sun Yat-sen Ophthalmology Center of Sun Yat-Sen University (Lin *et al.*, 2021) published an artificial intelligence model for diabetic retinopathy recognition in the international top issue *The Lancet Digital Health*, which can identify 14 common fundus based on fundus images disease, obtained the artificial intelligence software category III medical device product registration certificate issued by the State Food and Drug Administration.

Although the application of deep learning in the field of ophthalmic medical image analysis has been very common in recent years and has achieved great success, it still faces many challenges, mainly in the following aspects:

Deep learning technology needs to train models based on big data. However, in real life, due to factors such as data management, privacy restrictions, scarcity of data for rare diseases, and uneven distribution of different lesions, a large-scale standard medical data are established. Collection is very difficult. Therefore, many studies use training datasets of relatively homogeneous populations, and the characteristics of the lesions in the datasets are relatively single, which restricts the model learning and affects the final effect of the model. In addition, the training and testing of deep learning models using retinal images will be affected by many variable factors, such as differences in fundus image acquisition equipment, imaging quality, field of view, market width, and patient cooperation, which will all be affected to varying degrees. Influence the deep learning model for the pathological characteristics of different diseases, especially the learning of fine-grained pathological characteristics. Therefore, the improvement of ophthalmic image acquisition equipment and technology upgrades make the diagnosis methods of fundus diseases conform to the development of the times. At the same time, fundus image analysis based on artificial intelligence technology also requires researchers to make new attempts and explorations to achieve new breakthroughs.

1.4   The Main Content of This Book

On the basis of the predecessors, this book explores the implementation methods based on deep learning for the screening, diagnosis, and lesion detection and segmentation of several types of common fundus diseases with respect to the challenges and difficulties mentioned above. The problem of the limitation of the dataset mentioned in this book has spent a lot of manpower, material, and financial resources on the establishment and improvement of the dataset, and the new dataset is used for model training so that the model achieves excellent results. Part of the system has also been deployed to offline hospitals and has achieved excellent results in clinical applications.

The main content of this book includes the following: establishing and improving fundus disease datasets, including ROP, DR, and ultrawide-angle fundus image datasets; for ROP book, a network model based on feature aggregation operators is proposed, and the model is combined with cloud platforms for research and development of ROP automatic screening systems; in addition, the book also includes DR automatic diagnosis and grading models and systems based on transfer learning and integrated learning, macular edema (ME) lesion segmentation methods for optical coherence tomography (OCT) images, and a screening system for multiple fundus diseases based on ultrawide-angle fundus images.

Chapter 2

Automated Analysis for Retinopathy of Prematurity by Deep Neural Networks

Retinopathy of prematurity (ROP) is the leading cause of childhood blindness worldwide. Automated ROP detection system is urgent and it appears to be a safe, reliable, and cost-effective complement. Deep neural networks (DNNs) can directly learn abstract features from big data without the explicit knowledge of experts and yield impressive results. Automated ROP detection system using DNNs requires further assessment and validation to improve ROP care. In this study, automated ROP detection was divided into ROP identification and grading tasks. Two specific DNNs, i.e., Id-Net and Gr-Net, were designed for identification and grading tasks, respectively. To develop the DNNs, large-scale datasets of retinal fundus images were constructed by labeling the images of ROP screenings by clinical ophthalmologists. On the test dataset, the Id-Net achieved a sensitivity of 96.62% (95% CI, 92.29–98.89%) and a specificity of 99.32% (95% CI, 96.29–9.98%) for ROP identification while the Gr-Net attained sensitivity and specificity values of 88.46% (95% CI, 96.29–99.98%) and 92.31% (95% CI, 81.46–97.86%), respectively, on the ROP grading task. In another 552 cases, the developed DNN model outperformed some human experts. An automated ROP detection system called DeepROP was obtained by integrating the DNNs with a cloud computing platform. In a clinical setting, the sensitivity and specificity values of DeepROP for ROP identification were

11

84.91% (95% CI, 76.65–91.12%) and 96.90% (95% CI, 95.49–97.96%), respectively, whereas the corresponding measures for ROP grading were 93.33% (95% CI, 68.05–99.83%) and 73.63% (95% CI, 68.05–99.83%), respectively. The developed DeepROP system attained high sensitivity and specificity for automated ROP detection in retinal fundus images.

2.1 Methods

In this study, we developed an automated ROP screening system using DNN models. It could be used for telemedicine ROP screening and facilitate cooperation among hospitals. In this section, the methods to construct the ROP detection datasets, and develop and evaluate the DNN models as well as the automated ROP screening systems are presented.

2.1.1 *Image labeling*

First, a large set of retinal fundus images from the ROP screening of premature babies should be collected. During each ROP screening, several retinal fundus images are captured which are split into two sets according to the eyes since the healthy state of each eye could be different. Each set is defined as a case that is to be labeled independently.

The cases were labeled by four clinical ophthalmologists following the pipelines in Fig. 2.1. In the initial blind-reading phase, each case was annotated separately by three ophthalmologists. A case was annotated as "ROP" if ROP was found in any of its retinal fundus images; otherwise, it was annotated as "normal". The ROP case was then graded into "minor ROP" or "severe ROP" according to its severity. Therefore, two datasets were constructed: an identification dataset and a grading dataset. In the subsequent non-blind phase, the annotations were evaluated by another more experienced clinical ophthalmologist if the assigned labels varied among the initial experts. The fourth ophthalmologist dropped the cases if diagnoses were not faithful.

The labels, i.e., "normal", "minor ROP", and "severe ROP", used in this study were assigned not only based on the International

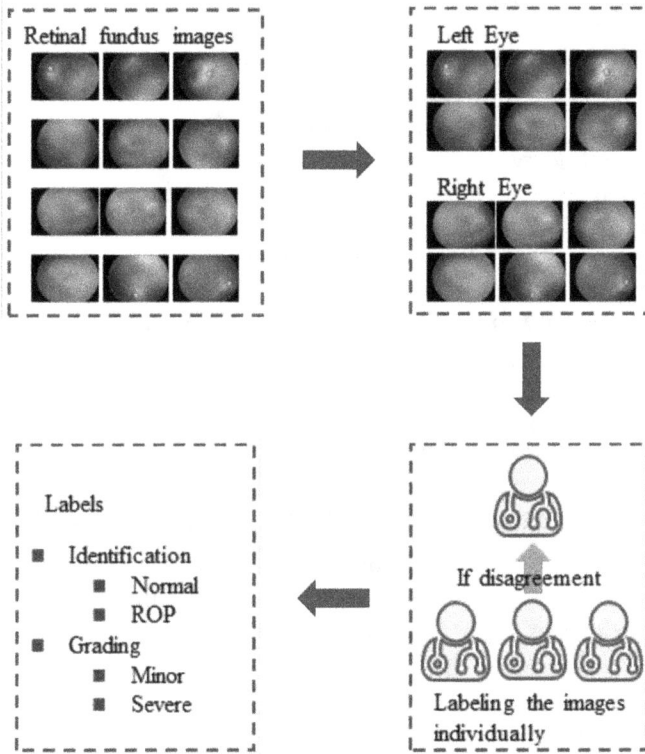

Fig. 2.1. The image labeling process.

Committee for the Classification of Retinopathy of Prematurity (ICROP) system (Moskowitz, 2016) but also based on the requirements of clinical treatment described in Cryotherapy for Retinopathy of Prematurity (CRYO-ROP) (Quinn, 2005) and Early Treatment ROP (ETROP) (Group *et al.*, 2003; Quinn, 2005). The identification labels, "normal" and "ROP", denote whether the clinical features of ROP are found in the retinal fundus images. The grading labels, "minor ROP" and "severe ROP", indicate the severity of the ROP disease. The clinical features of "minor ROP" are Zone II or III and stage 1 or 2, while the clinical features of "severe ROP" are threshold disease, type I, type II, or AP-ROP, and stage 4 or 5. The details of the definitions of the clinical features of ROP can be found in the literature (Group *et al.*, 2003; Moskowitz, 2016; Quinn, 2005).

2.1.2 *Deep neural networks*

ROP detection consists of two subtasks. One is an identification task, which aims to distinguish ROP cases from normal cases. The other is a grading task, where cases of ROP are classified into minor and severe. The two subtasks are binary classification problems in machine learning, which can be formulated as

$$F : X = \{x_i | i = 1, 2, \ldots, n\} \to y, \qquad (2.1)$$

where n is the number of images of case X and x_i is the i-th image. $y \in \{1, 2\}$ is the corresponding label of X. Our goal is to approximate the function F.

The methods in the literature (Worrall *et al.*, 2016; Brown *et al.*, 2018) cannot be applied directly to our work since the detection in this study was performed upon each case rather than each image independently. There are four challenges making it difficult for human eye as well as DNN models to identify and grade the ROP through the retinal fundus images: (1) The number of the images varies in different cases depending on the patient and the photographer. (2) Images of the retinal fundus are usually poor in quality because of motion blur and illumination artifacts. The color images are with significant appearance variations. (3) Only a few images in ROP cases contain the distinguished feature that determines ROP while the others are similar images between the different cases. (4) The feature that determines ROP is present in some very small local regions of the image.

To deal with the above problems, an ROP detection algorithm is developed by using deep convolutional neural networks (see Fig. 2.2). An identification network (Id-Net) and a grading network (Gr-Net) were developed to approximate the mapping for the aforementioned two subtasks, respectively. Id-Net and Gr-Net have similar network architecture (see Fig. 2.3). It was constructed by introducing a feature-binding block to the well-known Inception–BN (Ioffe and Szegedy, 2015) network, which delivered state-of-the-art performance in the large-scale image classification challenge "ImageNet".

The proposed Id-Net and Gr-Net consist of three blocks. The first is a feature extractor block, which is identical to the subnetwork from the input layer to the second Inception-B block in the

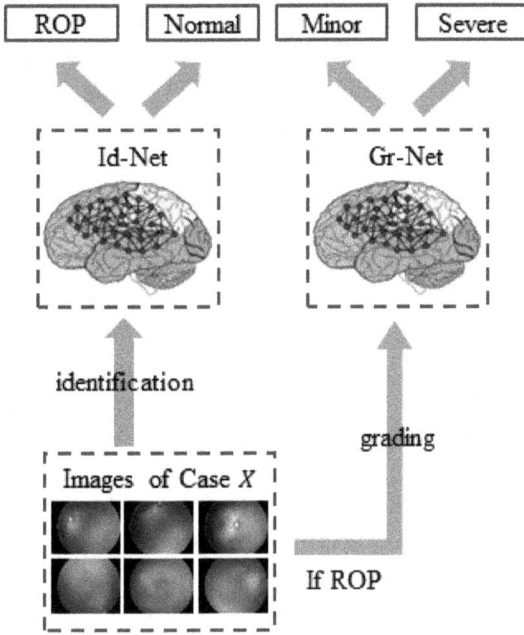

Fig. 2.2.   The workflow of ROP detection by using two DNNs. Case X was first identified by Id-Net and subsequently graded by Gr-Net if it was an ROP case.

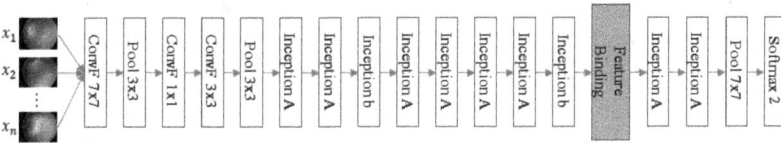

Fig. 2.3.   The architecture of the DNNs used in the algorithm. The feature-binding block was implemented by an element-wise max operation. The architectures of the Conv Factory, Inception A, and Inception B modules are identical to the corresponding modules in the Inception–BN (Ioffe and Szegedy, 2015) network.

Inception–BN (Ioffe and Szegedy, 2015) network. Given a case X, the feature extractor block takes each image x_i one by one and outputs the corresponding feature map s_i. The second block is the feature-binding block, which aims to bind the set of feature maps $S = \{s_i | i = 1, 2, \ldots, n\}$ into one feature map $S(X)$. The feature fusing method used in our networks is the max operation, defined by $S(X)^j = \max\{s_i^j | i = 1, 2, \ldots, n\}$, where s_i^j is the j-th element of the i-th feature map, and $S(X)^j$ is the j-th element of feature map

$S(X)$. The feature-binding block can reduce negative effects of the varying number of images in each case X and can enhance the feature maps of distinguishable images while suppressing similar images that are found in many cases belonging to different categories. The third block is the classification block, which consists of several convolution layers and a softmax layer. It learns deep abstract features from feature map $S(X)$ and maps the final feature into the corresponding label of the input case.

Id-Net and Gr-Net need to be trained on the large-scale dataset to obtain the network parameters. The training of a neural network refers to changing the parameters in it to improve network performance by deploying a learning algorithm, such as the backpropagation (BP) algorithm. The network performance is described by a cost function that measures the distance between the network's output and the real label. After training, the neural network is expected to produce an output that is close to the corresponding real label. The training processes of Id-Net and Gr-Net were identical except for the training dataset used. Id-Net was trained on the identification dataset, whereas the Gr-Net was trained on the grading dataset. The training process consisted of two phases. The first was offline pretraining. An Inception–BN network was trained on ImageNet. The learned parameters were used as the initial parameters of Id-Net and Gr-Net, which were then fine-tuned on the corresponding ROP dataset. Here, the retinal fundus images were resized from $1200 \times 1600 \times 3$ to $240 \times 320 \times 3$ and the values of the pixels were normalized into range $[-1, 1]$. Cross-entropy was used as cost function. The optimization method was Adadelta (Zeiler, 2012) with the default parameters $lr = 1.0$, $rho = 0.9$, and $eps = 1e - 06$. The proposed DNN models were implemented using TensorFlow (https://www.tensorflow.org) and the source code is available on GitHub at https://github.com/qmiwang/deeprop.

2.1.3 *Experts' comparisons*

To further evaluate the performance of the developed DNN models, the retinal fundus images captured during routine clinical ROP screenings in Jan. 2018 at Chengdu Women and Children's Central

Hospital were used to compare the DNN models' predictions with the diagnoses of three human experts.

Having developed a labeling system, we instructed three experts with adequate clinical experience in ROP detection to make a referral decision on each case using only the retinal fundus image independently. Given a case, the true label was given by the voting of the labels made by three experts. It means that the label of a given case is obtained by choosing the label given by at least two experts. The confusion table and error rate of the DNN model and the three experts were calculated by referring to the true labels. Furthermore, we computed the KAPPA values between the DNN model and the three experts, respectively.

2.1.4 *Testing of the DeepROP system under clinical settings*

The ROP detection algorithm was integrated into a cloud computing platform for automated ROP detection in images of the retinal fundus. The platform is called DeepROP. It can be used for telemedicine ROP screening and cooperation among hospitals. In general, the workflow consists of the following stages (see Fig. 2.4):

Step 1: Uploading images of the retinal fundus. In a hospital that has ROP screening devices, prematurely born infants undergo ROP screening programs. The photographer, doctor, or anyone who can obtain images of the retinal fundus can access the automated ROP detection platform and upload the images through a website.

Step 2: Automated ROP detection. The automated ROP detection platform saves the retinal fundus images and automatically divides them into two cases: images of the left eye and those of the right eye. Given a case, Id-Net takes the images as input and generates the ROP identification results. The detection process is complete if the given case is determined to be normal. Otherwise, Gr-Net is executed to determine the severity of ROP. Finally, an initial diagnostic report is generated automatically. This process does not require any human assistance. It eliminates the drawbacks stemming from a lack of adequately trained clinicians for ROP identification.

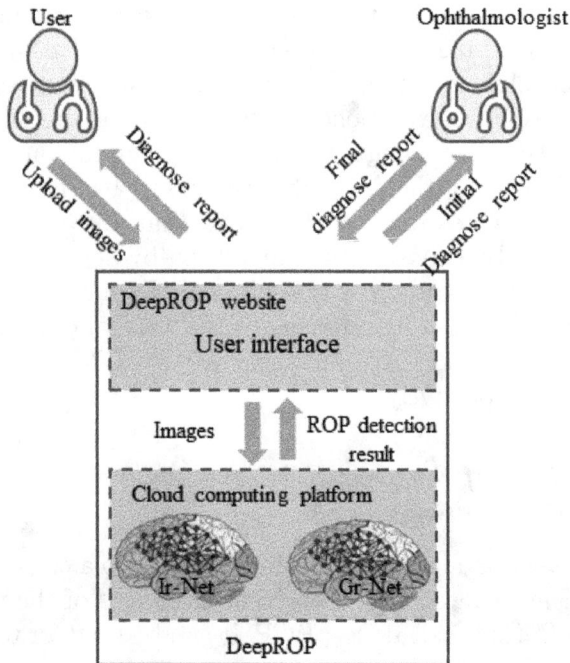

Fig. 2.4. The workflow of developed DeepROP system in the clinical test. The cloud-based platform consists of the proposed DNN models and the DeepROP website as the user interface.

Step 3: ROP expert evaluation. The diagnostic report contains a confidence score for the automated ROP detection platform. If the confidence score is below a threshold, the results should be evaluated by human experts. They can check the report online, and one report can be evaluated by several experts. Our cloud-based platform thus supports cooperation among hospitals for ROP diagnosis.

The website was assessed in six hospitals for routine ROP screening programs. The clinical ophthalmologist uploaded images captured during routine clinical ROP Screening programs without any data selection or preprocessing. The DeepROP system would generate the diagnosis automatically. By referring to the diagnosis by the clinical ophthalmologist as the standard label, the specificity and sensitivity of the model were presented.

2.2 Results

In this study, we constructed a large-scale ROP dataset of retinal fundus images and developed two DNN models for the detection of ROP. One is Id-Net which aims to distinguish the normal case from ROP case and the other is Gr-Net which classifies the ROP cases into either Minor ROP case or Severe ROP case. The two DNN models were trained and evaluated on the constructed dataset and then integrated into a cloud-based platform for automated ROP detection, which was assessed in the routine ROP screening in multiple hospitals in China.

2.2.1 *Large-scale ROP datasets*

We collected lots of images of ROP screenings from the Chengdu Women and Children's Central Hospital. Following the proposed image labeling method, there were 349 cases drop in the identification dataset and 222 cases drop in the grading task. The proposed datasets consist of three parts: developing data to build the DNN models, data for expert comparison, and data collected from the Web. The number of cases and images are listed in Table 2.1. The cases in developing data and data for expert comparison were collected from screenings of 869 infants. The summaries of the birth weights and gestation ages of the infants are presented in Fig. 2.5. As expected, most of them had low birth weights or were premature. There were

Table 2.1. Summaries of datasets used in this study.

| | | Identification Task | | | Grading Task | | | |
| | | Normal | | ROP | | Minor ROP | | Severe ROP | |
	#patients	#cases	#images	#cases	#images	#cases	#images	#cases	#images
Developing data	605	1484	7559	742	5967	260	1834	260	2305
Data for expert comparison	264	501	2068	51	293	31	173	20	120
Data from web	404	838	4251	106	657	91	565	15	92

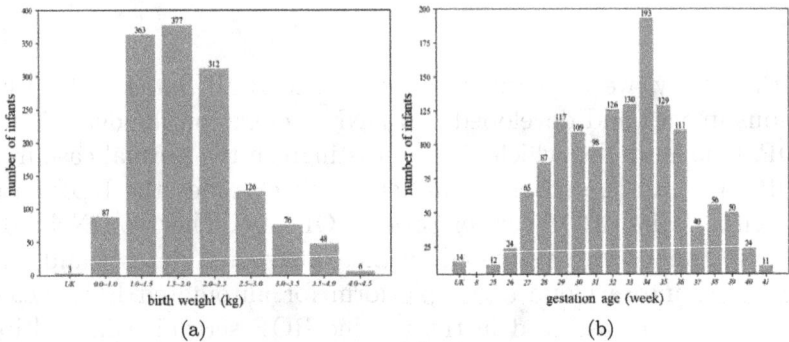

Fig. 2.5.   The distributions of birth weight and gestation ages of the infants. "UK" denotes the set of infants whose birth weights or gestation ages were not provided. (a) Each bar represents the number of sets of infants whose birth weights were in the given range. (b) Each bar represents the number of sets of infants whose gestation ages were within the given weeks.

Table 2.2.   Summaries of different datasets for ROP detection.

	Patients	Cases	Images	Labels
Canada [3]	35	347	1459	Normal/plus
London [3]	—	—	106	Normal/plus
Dataset [8]	—	—	77	Normal/plus/preplus
Ours	1273	3722	20,795	Normal/minor/severe

93 boys and 78 girls while the genders of other infants were unknown since they were not recorded during the ROP screening.

To the best of our knowledge, this is the largest dataset of images of the retinal fundus for ROP detection. A comparison of our dataset with published datasets is listed in Table 2.2. Our dataset was more heterogeneous as it contained images of more patients and more cases of ROP screening. It would be a good tutorial for ROP education because it ensures coverage of the various instances of different ROP severities. Furthermore, the scale of the dataset is key to the success of automated ROP grading methods, such as DNNs. The labels used in our dataset were designed according to the clinical treatment of ROP patients in Sichuan, China. It is thus more suitable for patients in China.

2.2.2 Performance of the model

To train and evaluate DNN models, the developing dataset was split randomly. 298 cases (149 normal and 149 ROP) and 104 cases (52 minor ROP and 52 severe ROP) were selected randomly from the developing dataset for evaluating the performance of Id-Net and Gr-Net, respectively. Other cases were used to train Id-Net and Gr-Net. To deal with the imbalance problems, during the training, we oversampled the classes with less cases to ensure the number of cases is the same in each task.

By referring to annotations provided by four ophthalmologists, the proportions of false positives and missed cases of the optimized DNNs were recorded. The results are presented in Fig. 2.6, Tables 2.3 and 2.4. In the identification task, the developed Id-Net distinguished normal cases from ROP cases with a sensitivity of 96.64% (95% CI, 92.34%–98.90%) and a specificity of 99.33% (95% CI, 96.32%–99.98%). The area under the ROC curve was 99.49%. Using Gr-Net, the algorithm provided ROP grading attained sensitivity and specificity values of 88.46% (95% CI, 76.56%–95.65%) and 92.31% (95% CI, 81.46%–97.86%), respectively. The area under the ROC curve was 95.08%.

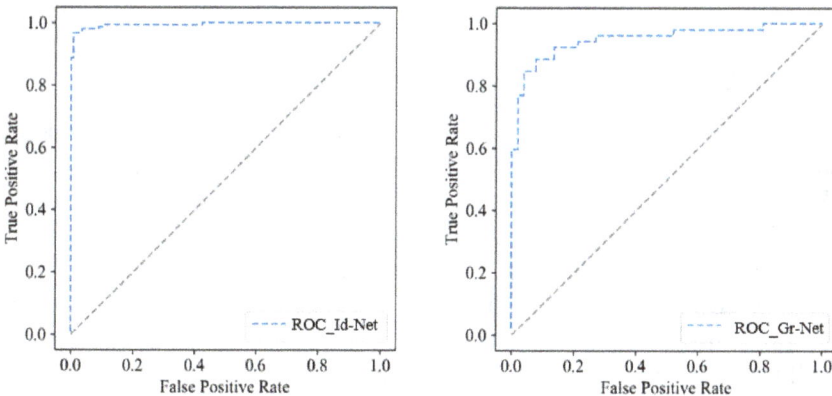

Fig. 2.6.   Receiver operating characteristic (ROC) curves of DNN models for identification task (left) and grading task (right).

Table 2.3. Confusion table of Id-Net for identification task.

		Predicted label	
		Normal	ROP
True label	Normal	148	1
	ROP	5	144

Table 2.4. Confusion table of Gr-Net for grading task.

		Predicted label	
		Minor ROP	Severe ROP
True label	Minor ROP	48	4
	Severe ROP	6	46

Table 2.5. Inter-rater KAPPA values.

	DNN models	Expert 1	Expert 2	Expert 3	Label
DNN model	1	0.34	0.70	0.70	0.68
Expert 1	0.34	1	0.32	0.42	0.53
Expert 2	0.70	0.32	1	0.69	0.80
Expert 3	0.70	0.42	0.69	1	0.89
Label	0.68	0.53	0.80	0.89	1

2.2.3 *Comparison of the model with human experts*

The datasets for expert comparison were the retinal fundus images captured during routine clinical ROP in January 2018 at Chengdu Women and Children's Central Hospital to compare the developed DNN's referral decisions with the decisions made by human experts. There are 2361 images of 552 cases from 264 patients. The distributions of the normal cases, minor ROP cases, and severe ROP cases are presented in Table 2.1.

The inter-rater KAPPA values among the DNN models and three experts are presented in Table 2.5. Furthermore, the confusion tables and error rates of the DNN models and the three experts are presented in Tables 2.6–2.9 and Fig. 2.7. The developed DNN models outperformed expert 1.

Table 2.6. The confusion table of the DNNs on the dataset used for the comparison of the model with experts.

		Predicted label		
		Normal	Minor	Severe
True label	Normal	487	11	3
	Minor	6	16	9
	Severe	2	1	17

Table 2.7. The confusion table of expert 1 on the dataset used for the comparison of the model with experts. The confusion table of expert 1 on the dataset used for the comparison of the model with experts.

		Predicted label		
		Normal	Minor	Severe
True label	Normal	499	0	2
	Minor	15	16	0
	Severe	5	15	0

Table 2.8. The confusion table of expert 2 on the dataset used for the comparison of the model with experts.

		Predicted label		
		Normal	Minor	Severe
True label	Normal	492	9	0
	Minor	1	20	10
	Severe	0	0	20

Table 2.9. The confusion table of expert 3 on the dataset used for the comparison of the model with experts.

		Predicted label		
		Normal	Minor	Severe
True label	Normal	489	12	0
	Minor	0	31	0
	Severe	0	0	20

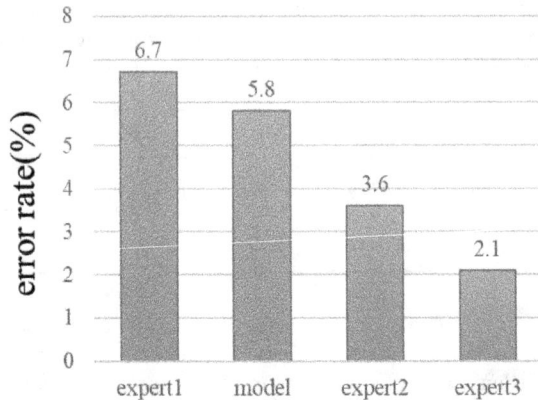

Fig. 2.7.   The error rates of the experts and the developed DNN model.

Furthermore, the average time per case used by the DNNs is around 2 seconds while it is around 30–60 seconds for human experts. The detection prediction by the DNN models is very efficient.

2.2.4   *DeepROP website and clinical test*

The proposed ROP detection algorithm was integrated with a cloud computing platform for automated ROP detection and report generation by the proposed networks, sample search and download, report evaluation, and interaction between patients and ophthalmologists.

The website was assessed in six hospitals for routine ROP screening programs, including Chengdu Women and Children's Central Hospital, Xin Hua Hospital Affiliated to Shanghai Jiao Tong University School of Medicine, Ya An People's Hospital, People's Hospital of De Yang City, Affiliated Hospital of North Sichuan Medical College, and Affiliated Hospital of Southwest Medical University. The clinical ophthalmologist uploaded images captured during routine clinical ROP screening programs without any data selection or preprocessing. The developed DNN models achieved good performance. From March 3 to December 28, 2017, 472 ROP screenings were conducted on 404 infants in Chengdu Women and Children's Central Hospital. The clinical ophthalmologist uploaded images from these 472 screenings to the website. DeepROP automatically divided the images into 944 cases according to the eye. For each case, it made two predictions for identification and grading, respectively, and generated

Table 2.10. Summaries of the performance of DNNs used in DeepROP website in clinical test.

	Id-Net	Gr-Net
Sensitivity	84.91% (95% CI, 76.65–91.12%)	93.33% (95% CI, 68.05–99.83%)
Specificity	96.90% (95% CI, 95.49–97.96%)	73.63% (95% CI, 68.05–99.83%)
Accuracy	95.55% (95% CI, 94.03–96.77%)	76.42% (95% CI, 67.18–84.12%)

an initial diagnostic report that was evaluated by a clinical ophthalmologist. The ophthalmologist edited the report if his/her diagnosis was inconsistent with the initial report by DeepROP. For comparison, the diagnosis by the clinical ophthalmologist was referred to as the standard label. The ophthalmologist's diagnosis and DeepROP predictions were then recorded. The performance of DeepROP is shown in Table 2.10.

2.3 Discussions

Automated ROP grading algorithms are desirable for ROP screening and treatment. Dataset plays a crucial role in the training of automated ROP grading algorithms. In general, a dataset used for DNNs must contain a large number of images of ROP screenings that cover various ROP features and different severities, and have been captured from an adequately large number of patients to reduce the individual effect and avoid the overfitting of the learning algorithm to some specific feature. Otherwise, the performance of the learning algorithm worsens when applied to new images of ROP screening. The datasets constructed in this study are advantageous in terms of the above properties over other datasets. Moreover, both the identification dataset and grading dataset were provided, which enabled the process to grade cases of ROP for accurate treatment rather than simply identify ROP.

The results showed that DNNs can be trained using large-scale datasets, without the need to specify features by experts, to automatically detect ROP in images of the retinal fundus with high sensitivity and accuracy. Compared with human experts with adequate clinical experience in ROP diagnosis, the developed DNNs obtained comparable performance and made the detection prediction very efficient. Further, it provides the same diagnosis on a given image every time, which is difficult for a human ophthalmologist. Multiple DNN models can be trained and integrated to simulate the consultation of several experts as well. This will be tested in our future work. Furthermore, the proposed method in this study is more suitable to be deployed in the automated ROP screening system than the methods in the other literatures because our method detects the ROP per case no matter how many images there are.

The clinical setting test highlighted the impressive performance of the DeepROP platform. Results suggest that while ROP identification worked very well prospectively, the ROP grading does not do so well. Maybe there are two reasons. One is that the features between "minor ROP" cases and "severe ROP" cases are less distinguishable than the features between "Normal" cases and "ROP" cases. The other is that the number of cases used to develop the Gr-Net is smaller than the number of cases used to develop the Id-Net so that the generalization performance of the Gr-Net is poorer than that of the Id-Net. The clinical setting test is an important step in telemedicine ROP screening programs and multi-hospital collaboration for several reasons. First, it enables ROP prescreening and evaluation of patients in non-specialized hospitals. Second, it breaks the bottleneck of data usage due to the isolation of data in individual hospitals and accelerates the process of collecting a large-scale dataset for fine-grained ROP grading. Third, the cloud-based platform can collect new data, which will increase the coverage of ROP features, and improve the ROP detection algorithm. For example, in the Web-based test in this study, 4908 images of 944 cases of 404 infants were collected in 10 months. The size of those data items was larger than published datasets.

The limitations of our work lie in three aspects. First, the number of "severe ROP" cases is not enough to ensure the generalization performance in the clinical test. Second, the developed system can only evaluate the severity of ROP. In future work, we plan to collect more data and grade ROP in more fine-grained classes, such as the "plus-disease", "stage", and "zone". Third, an open question is whether the predictions of the cloud platform will influence the diagnoses of ophthalmologists in comparison with clinical testing without the platform. More attention should be paid to test the platform more widely in future.

Chapter 3

DeepROP: An Automated ROP Screening System

Retinopathy of prematurity (ROP) is a retinal vasoproliferative disorder disease principally observed in infants born prematurely with low birth weight. ROP is an important cause of childhood blindness. Although automatic or semi-automatic diagnosis of ROP has been conducted, most previous studies have focused on "plus" disease, which is indicated by abnormalities of retinal vasculature. Few studies have reported methods for identifying the "stage" of ROP disease. Deep neural networks have achieved impressive results in many computer vision and medical image analysis problems, raising expectations that it might be a promising tool in automatic diagnosis of ROP. In this chapter, convolutional neural networks (CNNs) with novel architecture are proposed to recognize the existence and severity of ROP disease per-examination. The severity of ROP is divided into mild and severe cases according to the disease progression. The proposed architecture consists of two subnetworks connected by a feature aggregate operator. The first subnetwork is designed to extract high-level features from images of the fundus. These features from different images in an examination are fused by the aggregate operator and then used as the input for the second subnetwork to predict its class. A large dataset imaged by RetCam 3 is used to train and evaluate the model. The high classification accuracy in the experiment demonstrates the effectiveness of the proposed architecture for recognizing ROP disease.

3.1   Retinopathy of Prematurity

As the primary cause of childhood blindness, Retinopathy of prematurity (ROP) is an eye disease that occurs frequently in infants with low birth weight and premature birth (Tasman *et al.*, 2006). ROP was initially known as Retrolental Fibroplasia (RLF) and originally observed by Terry in the 1940s (Terry, 1942). Nowadays, it is widely accepted that ROP is closely associated with excessive oxygen use. During gestation, the development of blood vessels begins in the fourth month of gestation, reaching the retinal periphery before birth (Roth, 1977). For premature infants, relative hyperoxia in the extrauterine environment and the continuous supply of oxygen can slow down the growth rate of retinal vasculature and lead to tissue hypoxia. Retinal neovascularization may then develop at the joint between vascular and avascular areas, producing scar tissue causing retinal detachment through retraction (Chen and Smith, 2007).

As the harm caused by this potentially blinding disorder has become clear, an international group formed by ROP experts published a detailed classification guideline in 1984 and 1987 to facilitate the development of clinical treatment and improve understanding of the condition (Committee for the Classification of Retinopathy of Prematurity, 1984; ICROP Committee for Classification of Late Stages ROP, 1988). First, the guideline defined three zones to better describe the location of the illness in ROP with each zone centered on the optic disc. Second, five stages of ROP and a type of ancillary illness called "plus" were proposed. Symptoms of Stages 1–5 are listed in Table 3.1. Plus disease occurs in conjunction with ROP and is characterized by increased dilation and tortuosity in retinal vessels. Figure 3.1 shows images of the fundus in normal development and at Stages 2 and 3 of ROP. According to the reported recommendations (Good *et al.*, 2004), any stage of ROP with plus in Zone I, Stage 3 of ROP without plus in Zone I, and Stage 2 or 3 with plus in Zone II require early treatment. There was no appropriate treatment for ROP until the 1980s and 1990s when laser photocoagulation and cryotherapy were shown to be effective methods for preventing blindness in infants (Chen and Smith, 2007). Although these therapies can reduce the incidence of blindness in infants, they also impact patients' visual acuity. Early diagnosis and timely treatment can help reduce the adverse outcomes and vision loss (Campbell *et al.*, 2016).

Table 3.1. Symptoms of Stage 1 to 5 of ROP

Stage	Symptoms
1	A thin demarcation line separates vascularized and avascular areas
2	Line in Stage 1 evolves to a ridge
3	Extraretinal fibrovascular proliferation in the ridge
4	Partial retinal detachment
5	Total retinal detachment

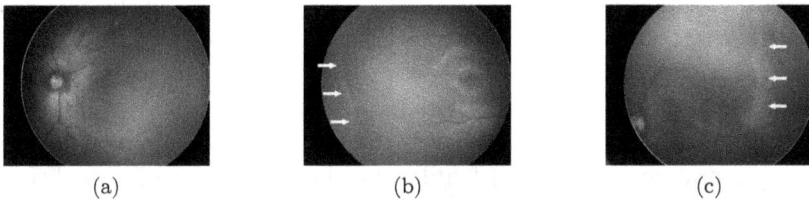

(a)   (b)   (c)

Fig. 3.1. Fundus photographs imaged by RetCam 3. From left to right are normal, Stage 2, and Stage 3 of ROP, respectively. There is an obvious ridge at the junction between vascularized and avascular retina in both Stages 2 and 3 of ROP. In Stage 3, fibrovascular proliferation can be observed from the ridge into the vitreous.

Diagnosis of ROP requires inspecting the fundus of premature infants from different views using imaging systems like RetCam 3, which is a digital retinal camera with high image quality. The imaging data are then interpreted by experienced ophthalmologists to determine the presence of the symptoms of ROP or plus disease described above. However, the diagnosis can be challenging for several reasons. First, developing countries such as China and India have an insufficient number of qualified ophthalmologists to match the number of premature infants (Yau *et al.*, 2015; Shah *et al.*, 2016). In these countries, there is a pressing need for ophthalmologists. Second, the quality of imaging is affected by many factors (e.g., focus, illumination, and eyes' movement). Third, the classification guidelines provide only qualitative signs rather than quantitative descriptions. Thus, clinical assessment mainly depends on the ophthalmologist's subjective interpretation of the symptoms (Aslam *et al.*, 2009). As a result, there exists disagreement in diagnoses between different experts assessing the same examination. This uncertainty has been reported when diagnosing the presence of plus disease and the stage of ROP (Gschließer *et al.*, 2015; Chiang *et al.*, 2007). To assist ophthalmologists in the diagnosis of ROP, a number of computer-aided diagnosis systems have been proposed. Most of the proposed systems have focused on detecting plus disease, which is an illness that co-occurs with ROP that can be quantified (Worrall *et al.*, 2016). However, few of them focused on the automated stages classification of ROP.

In this study, a novel methodology based on deep neural networks is proposed to automatically recognize ROP in fundus images. Assessment of ROP is accomplished in two steps. The first step is designed to recognize whether ROP disease is present. If ROP is recognized, the second step is to assess the severity of the disease. Both steps are required to analyze examination data, which involve variable number of images in different views. This recognition method faces several challenges: (1) Unlike the characteristics of plus disease indicated by the dilation and tortuosity of posterior veins, the stage of ROP is characterized by the demarcation line between vascularized and avascular areas. The locations and shapes of the lines in the fundus vary significantly in each examination. (2) A massive amount of annotated data is required to learn the features of ROP from the data. However, the datasets in current ROP-related researches cannot meet this requirement. (3) Each examination of the fundus contains a number of images with different views. To obtain the ROP recognition result, the model must jointly analyze multiple images in an examination.

To address the first challenge, convolutional neural networks (CNNs) with a powerful abstract ability are used. CNNs have been widely applied in computer vision-related problems and have been shown to learn high-level features directly from data. Meanwhile, transfer learning is used in the work to facilitate the training phase. Transfer learning is an effective method to train the very deep CNNs when the target dataset is small. It has been widely used in medical imaging applications and performs better than models trained from scratch (Tajbakhsh *et al.*, 2016). To solve the second challenge, a large-scale dataset annotated by some experienced clinical ophthalmologists is used. To our best knowledge, the training dataset used in this study is larger than that of the previous ROP-related studies by an order of magnitude. The large dataset contributes to learn the disease-related characteristics in CNNs and reduces the

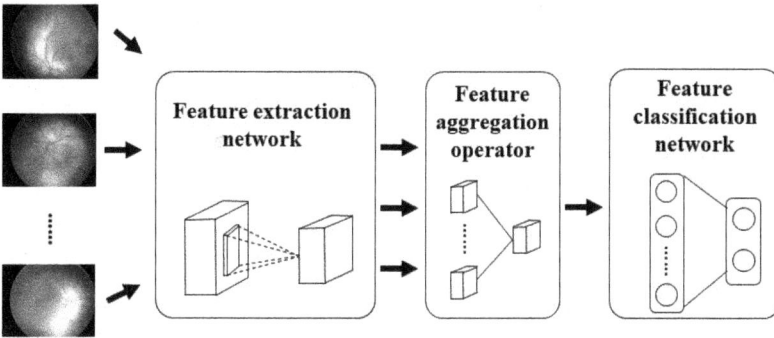

Fig. 3.2. The proposed architecture with two subnetworks for recognizing of ROP. The input is multiple fundus images of an examination. The first subnetwork is used to extract features in multiple images in an examination and the second one is used to classify the ROP disease. The extracted features from the multiple images in first subnetwork are aggregated before fed to the second subnetwork.

overfitting. To address the third challenge, a novel architecture of CNNs is proposed. Two subnetworks are included in the model: the first is designed to extract features from multiple images in an examination and the second is for classification. To jointly analyze the extracted features, an aggregate operator is used for binding features from the first subnetwork. The architecture of the proposed model is shown in Fig. 3.2. Several architectures of CNNs pretrained on ImageNet are explored, including the Visual Geometry Group (VGG) (Simonyan and Zisserman, 2014), Inception (Szegedy *et al.*, 2015; Ioffe and Szegedy, 2015), and Residual Networks (ResNets) (He *et al.*, 2016a,b).

This study makes several new contributions:

(i) A large dataset labeled by some experienced clinical ophthalmologists is used for automatically diagnosing ROP. The training dataset is larger than that of the previous ROP-related studies by an order of magnitude.

(ii) A novel ROP recognition architecture is proposed. The architecture contains two subnetworks which aim to extract and classify high-level features in a data-driven manner.

(iii) Feature aggregation operator is used to bind the features from different images in an examination. CNNs using the operator have superior accuracy compared with other state-of-the-art methods.

(iv) Two tasks are performed in this study, including recognition of the existence and severity of ROP. The classification and visualization results revealed the proposed architecture successfully learned the characteristics of ROP, providing a potentially useful tool to aid clinicians in diagnosing ROP disease.

3.2   Related Works

In this section, an overview of previous studies using traditional methods for ROP diagnosis is presented, followed by a brief introduction to deep neural networks and their application in ROP.

3.2.1   *Traditional methods for diagnosis of ROP*

The vast majority of automated or semi-automated methods for ROP diagnosis are focused on the recognition of plus disease, which is important for identifying infants with severe ROP disease. Since the existence and severity of plus disease are defined by the abnormality of vessels, most of these methods have attempted to measure statistics of vessels in fundus, such as diameter and tortuosity. Typically, three main steps are involved as follows: (a) vessel's segmentation, (b) measurement of the vessel's diameter (thickness), and (c) measurement of the vessel's tortuosity (Aslam *et al.*, 2009). The segmentation step requires accurate identification of the vascular tree from the retinal image, and the following two steps are based on the segmented vessels. Combined with these three steps, many computer-aided systems (CAD) have been proposed to assist ophthalmologists in improving diagnostic accuracy of ROP.

For example, a system called "ROPTool" has been proposed (Wallace *et al.*, 2007) to assist ophthalmologists in diagnosing plus disease. Using this system, operators first determine the area containing the vessels to be analyzed, which enables the system to track the vessels automatically using the "ridge/valley traversal" method (Aylward and Bullitt, 2002). To ameliorate overestimation, tortuosity was calculated as the total length of the vessel divided by the generated smooth curve instead of a straight line. Dilation was calculated by the average of the width over its length, divided by the area of the optic nerve. Based on the calculated values, operators can diagnose the existence of plus disease in a more quantitative way. "i-ROP" (Ataer-Cansizoglu *et al.*, 2015) was a system designed to grade plus disease into three types: normal, preplus, and plus. Principal spanning forest algorithm (Bas *et al.*, 2012) was used to extract the vessels. It goes a step further beyond "ROPTool", using 11 indices to quantify the tortuosity and dilation, including cumulative tortuosity index (CTI), integrated curvature (IC), integrated squared curvature (ISC), etc.

Although traditional methods have been found to aid diagnosis of ROP, there remain several challenges. Most to be solved, the precision of the measurement heavily relies on the vessel segmentation, meaning that errors in segmentation may be amplified in subsequent measurements. For measuring the diameter and tortuosity of the segmented vessels, the location of measurement and the effects of magnification differences may also impact the results [Aslam *et al.* (2009)].

3.2.2 *Deep neural networks for diagnosis of ROP*

Deep neural networks (Krizhevsky *et al.*, 2012; Simonyan and Zisserman, 2014) have received much interest in the field of machine learning. Two types of neural networks, including feed forward neural networks (FNNs) (Rumelhart *et al.*, 1986; LeCun *et al.*, 1998) and recurrent neural networks (RNNs) (Williams and Zipser, 1989; Yi and Tan, 2004; Yi, 2010; Wang *et al.*, 2017), have been heavily studied during the last decades. Since 2012, when AlexNet (Krizhevsky *et al.*, 2012) won the ILSVRC-2012 competition (Deng *et al.*, 2009), many important breakthroughs in computer vision have been achieved using deep neural networks. Several critical factors contribute to these achievements, including novel network architecture (Wang *et al.*, 2017; Simonyan and Zisserman, 2014; Szegedy *et al.*, 2015; He *et al.*, 2016b), powerful computation ability by utilizing graphics processing units (GPUs), and large-scale annotated datasets. Compared with traditional classification methods using handcraft features, it extracts different levels of features from low to high as the networks go deeper in a data-driven manner. Numerous studies have explored deep neural networks in a range of medical image analysis applications, including mitosis detection (Albarqouni *et al.*, 2016), lymph node detection (Shin *et al.*, 2016), lung pattern classification (Anthimopoulos *et al.*, 2016), and breast cancer classification (Carneiro *et al.*, 2017).

A recent study used an ImageNet pretrained GoogLeNet to classify the existence of plus disease in ROP (Worrall *et al.*, 2016), constituting the first attempt to use deep neural networks to diagnose plus disease. Two types of classification tasks were explored in the study, including the per-image and per-examination classifications. In the per-image classification, the researchers fine-tuned the convolutional kernel in the 9th inception block along the last fully connected layer. Based on the per-image classification, the researchers also proposed a per-examination classifier by assuming the Beta distribution prior over the probability that an examination is diagnosed with plus disease. Both the per-image and per-examination classifiers have superior performance than those of previous methods, demonstrating that CNNs may provide a promising tool for diagnosing ROP. Meanwhile, the visualization results revealed that CNNs have successfully learned the abnormalities in vessels correlated to plus disease.

The main characteristic in the ROP recognition is that there are variable number of fundus images in an examination. To solve this problem, Worrall *et al.* (2016) assumed the Beta distribution prior in per-examination classification. However, the assumption of Beta distribution is unfavorable in the generalization of the learned classifier because the parameters α and β in Beta distribution can't be tuned by the gradient-based optimization method.

According to previous study Good *et al.* (2004), besides plus disease, the stage of ROP is an important factor indicating whether early treatment is needed. In this study, a novel architecture based on the neural network model is proposed to identify ROP disease in per-examination manner. Unlike Worrall *et al.*'s method (Worrall *et al.*, 2016), the proposed model learns to recognize ROP directly from the data, instead of using a predefined assumption. The recognition is accomplished in two steps. The first step is to classify the existence of the ROP disease, and the second is to identify its severity. The proposed model has been trained and evaluated on a dataset of 2668 examinations, which is larger than the data in previous studies by an order of magnitude. To our best knowledge, this study is the first attempt to use a large dataset to recognize the existence and severity of ROP using deep neural networks.

3.3 Data and Methodology

In this section, the used dataset is first described in detail. The characteristics of the dataset provide a better understanding of the task. Then, the proposed model used in the two-step classification tasks is illustrated, including the architecture of networks and the feature aggregation operator.

3.3.1 *Data*

Before the data are used to train and evaluate the proposed model, three steps are needed: data imaging, data annotation, and data partition. The first step acquires fundus images in examinations, and the second annotates the examinations by experienced ophthalmologists. The annotated examinations are then partitioned into training, validation, and testing datasets in the third step. These three steps are described in detail in the following sections.

Data Imaging: Images of the fundus are obtained using RetCam 3 from the Chengdu Women and Children's Central Hospital (WCCH) from 2014 to 2017. The RetCam 3 can only capture one fixed view of the fundus at a time. To observe the fundus thoroughly, the operator typically takes multiple images of the fundus of the infant's eye in an examination. An examination of the left eye in Stage 2 of ROP is presented in Fig. 3.3. In this examination, the ridge in the fundus can be observed in (d) and (f). In this study, 2017 examinations are collected and 349 examinations are excluded in the annotation phase, which yield the final 2668 examinations from 720 infants. Each examination contains a variable number of images per eye. The resolution of the image is 1600 × 1200. The number of images per examination, gestation age, and birth weight are plotted as histograms in Fig. 3.4. The number of images per examination varies from 2 to 26, and the most frequently occurring number of images is 5. The gestation ages vary from 25 to 41 weeks, with a mean value of 32 weeks. 45% of the infants' gestation age is under 32 weeks. The maximum, minimum,

(a)   (b)   (c)

(d)   (e)   (f)

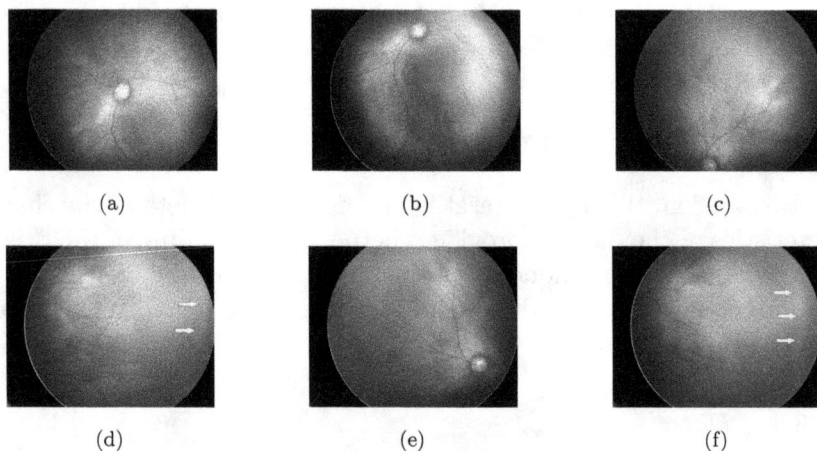

Fig. 3.3.   Multiple fundus images from different shooting angles in an examination of the left eye. An obvious ridge can be seen in Fig. 3.3(d) and Fig. 3.3(f) at the marked arrows, while Figs. 3.3(a)–3.3(c) and Fig. 3.3(e) appeared normal from visual inspection.

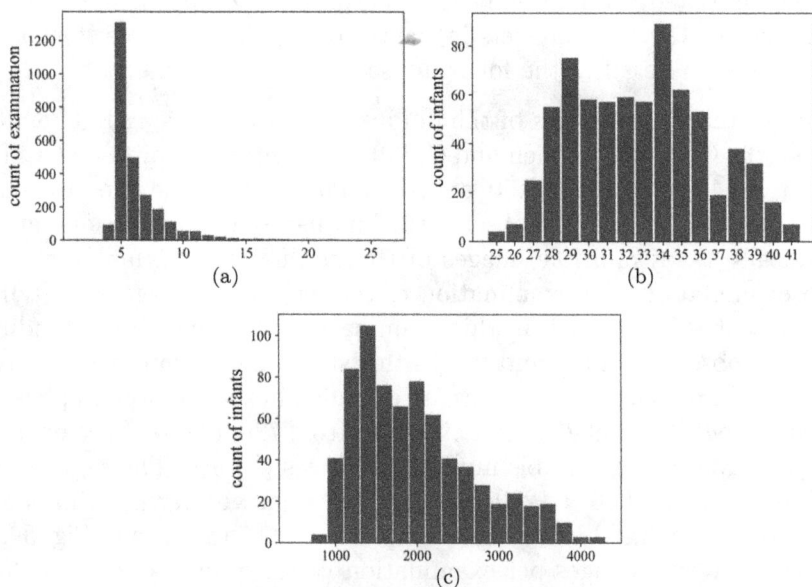

Fig. 3.4.   Histograms of the number of images per examination, gestation age, and birth weight. (a) Number of images in examinations, (b) examined infant's gestation age, and (c) examined infant's birth weight.

and mean birth weights are 4250, 700, and 1994 grams, respectively. 32% of the infants' birth weight is less than 1500 grams.

Data Annotation: The reference standard of the annotation complies with the symptoms described in Table 3.1. The process of the annotation is split into two phases: first, the ophthalmologists annotated examinations into normal and ROP types, followed by annotation of the severity of ROP. Both the two phases are annotated by three experienced ophthalmologists from the department of ophthalmology at Sichuan Academy of Medical Sciences and Sichuan Provincial People's Hospital. One of the annotators is the chief physician who has more than ten years of clinical experience in ROP. The other two annotators are both doctors who have over five years of clinical experience. In the first phase, the examinations with the consistent labels among the three ophthalmologists are picked out. The intersection process can minimize the subjective bias and reduce the risks caused by carelessness. Based on the examinations annotated as ROP in the first phase, the second phase requires the ophthalmologists to identify these examination stages. Similar to the two previous studies (Gschließer *et al.*, 2015; Bolón-Canedo *et al.*, 2015), a high diagnosis variability was observed among experts due to the subjective assessment. To ameliorate the potential effects of the bias, only the examinations with consistent labels among the three ophthalmologists are used. The quadratic-weighted kappa scores between the three ophthalmologists in the two annotation phases are shown in Fig. 3.5. It can be seen that the first two ophthalmologists have higher agreement than the third ophthalmologist in both annotation phases.

According to the annotation results, a high level of data imbalance is observed, where most ROP data are in Stages 2 and 3. There are relatively few ROP data in Stages 1, 4, and 5. There are two potential explanations for this imbalance: (1) The demarcation line separates the avascular and vascularized areas in both Stages 1 and 2, although the line is wider in Stage 2. These relative differences are determined subjectively, and the ophthalmologists tended to annotate them as Stage 2. (2) In Stages 4 and 5, retinal detachment can be observed. This phenomenon is rarely found in the current dataset because effective intervention will be carried out before the disease becomes severe. To solve the problem of imbalance, the ROP data

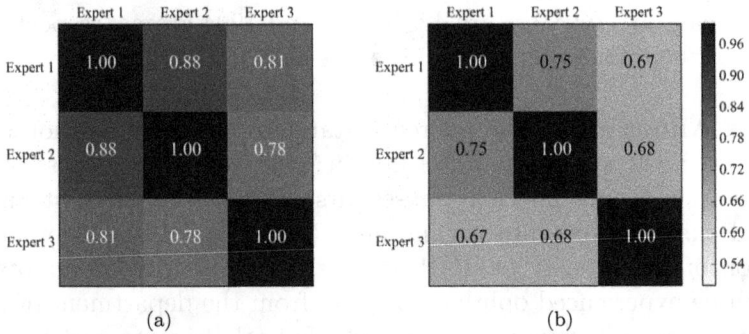

Fig. 3.5. The quadratic-weighted kappa score between the three ophthalmologists. (a) and (b) Represent the first and second annotations phases, respectively.

Table 3.2. Dataset used for training, evaluation, and testing the model.

	Normal	ROP	Mild	Severe
Train set	1184	884	225	241
Validation set	150	150	50	50
Test set	150	150	50	50
Total	1484	1184	325	341

are further divided into mild and severe cases according to the phase of the stage. Stages 1 and 2 are classified as mild, while Stages 3, 4, and 5 are classified as severe. This type of grading is consistent with the previous study (Committee for the Classification of Retinopathy of Prematurity, 1984; Ricard *et al.*, 2017), in which Stage 3 is an important phase between the growth of the demarcation line and the detachment of the retina. The last row in Table 3.2 shows the number of annotated examinations. There are 2668 identified examinations from 720 infants, including 1484 and 1184 examinations in normal and ROP, respectively. It should be noted that only examinations with consistent labels among the three annotators are included in the table, so the sum of mild and severe ROP cases is less than 1184.

Data Partition: The dataset used for training, evaluation, and testing the model is split in random and shown in the first three rows in Table 3.2. In the classification of normal and ROP, 150 examinations of normal and ROP are used as the validation and test dataset, respectively. The examinations on the left are used as training data.

In the classification of mild and severe ROP, 50 examinations of mild and severe cases are used as the validation and test datasets, and the remaining ROP examinations are used as training data.

3.3.2 *Methodology*

The inputs of our model are the annotated dataset $D = \{x_{i,j}, y_j; i = 1, \ldots, \tilde{N}, j = 1, \ldots, M\}$ containing M instances of examination, with corresponding labels. $x_{i,j} \in \mathbb{R}^{w \times h \times c}$, where w, h, and c denote the width, height, and channels of the fundus images, and i, j denote the i-th image in j-th examination. The $\tilde{N}$ varied from j since each examination could contain different numbers of fundus images. The goal is to learn a robust model $f(x, y; \theta)$ parameterized with θ, which maps the input image space $\mathcal{X}$ to the target space $\mathcal{Y}$.

Architecture of Networks: The model explored in this work is based on the CNNs. Three types of layers are typically included in CNNs: convolutional, pooling, and fully connected layers. In the convolutional layers, the parameters to learn are the kernels that connect with the input locally. The convolutional operation for single channel can be formulated as follows:

$$z_{v,u}^{l+1} = \sum_{p=0}^{P_l-1} \sum_{q=0}^{Q_l-1} \sum_{k=0}^{K_l-1} w_{p,q,k}^l \cdot a_{v+p,u+q,k}^l, \qquad (3.1)$$

where P, Q, and K denote the dimensions of the kernel and the lower-case letters denote the cursor in the kernel. v and u denote the spatial location of the output z^{l+1}. The shared kernel w^l convolves the input a^l along its dimensions of width and height to obtain the output. Then, a nonlinear activation function F is applied to z^{l+1},

$$a^{l+1} = F\left(z^{l+1}\right). \qquad (3.2)$$

Pooling is another important layer in CNNs, aiming to reduce the dimensionality of the inputs, thus decreasing the computational complexity. Two types of pooling are commonly used, including the max and mean pooling. In the pooling operation, the filter with fixed size slides over the spatial dimensions of input feature maps in a certain stride. During each slide process, the max or mean is calculated when max or mean pooling is used, respectively. The fully connected layer usually appears at the bottom of the CNNs. Unlike locally connected convolutional layers, each neuron in the fully connected layer has connections with all the neurons in the upper layer.

Fine-tuning with pretrained networks has been proven as an effective method for training CNNs. The pretraining of CNNs denotes the use of another dataset (e.g., ImageNet) to train a model parameterized with $\tilde{\boldsymbol{\theta}}$ by minimizing the loss function. Then, the parameters in the pretrained model are used to initialize the model $f(\boldsymbol{x}, \boldsymbol{y}; \boldsymbol{\theta})$ in the current task. In this study, several ImageNet pretrained networks are explored, including VGG (Simonyan and Zisserman, 2014), Inception (Szegedy *et al.*, 2015), and Residual Networks (He *et al.*, 2016b). The VGG network is stacked with multiple convolutional layers with very small kernel (3×3) and max pooling. The VGG network shows that the very small kernels are efficient for constructing CNNs. Inception is a kind of module that consists of max pooling and convolutional layer with the kernel size of 1×1, 3×3, and 5×5. To save computational resources, 1×1 convolutions are adhered to max pooling, 3×3, and 5×5 convolutions. The intuition behind the Inception module is to let the model itself learn the optimal structure among the different kinds of operations. To overcome the difficulties in training very deep CNNs, residual network has proposed another type of module that is composed of the residual and cross-layer shortcut connection. The module can be formulated as $\boldsymbol{a}^{l+1} = F^l(\boldsymbol{a}^l) + \boldsymbol{a}^l$, where $F^l(\boldsymbol{a}^l)$ and $\boldsymbol{a}^l$ denote the residual and shortcut connections, respectively.

Feature Aggregate Operator: Unlike traditional image classification task that the input to CNNs is a single image, the input in the ROP recognition is an examination containing $\tilde{N}$ variable images. This requires the model to make decisions based on multiple images. Consider the examination of ROP shown in Fig. 3.3; misdiagnose will happen when the model extracts features only from the image in Figs. 3.3(a)–3.3(c), or Fig. 3.3(e). To fully utilize the information in each image of an examination, the model should learn to aggregate features from all of those images. Then, the model is supposed to complete the recognition with the use of the aggregated features. However, *how* and *where* to aggregate features are two problems that should be solved. *How* represents the strategies used to aggregate the features. This is critically important for the model's accurate recognition because the disease-related characteristics may only appear in some of the images in an examination. *Where* denotes the aggregate location in the model. This is another major factor since it is unclear which is the optimal abstract level of the disease-related characteristics.

For the problem of *how*, inspired by the aggregation strategies used in fusing the spatial and temporal features (Feichtenhofer *et al.*, 2016), *max* and *mean* feature aggregate operators are explored in this study. The *max* and *mean* operators compute the max and average values of the $\tilde{N}$ features at the same spatial location, respectively. They can be formulated as

$$\tilde{a}_j^l = \max_{i \in [1,\tilde{N}_j]} a_i^l, \tag{3.3}$$

and

$$\tilde{a}_j^l = \frac{1}{\tilde{N}_j} \sum_{i=1}^{\tilde{N}_j} a_i^l, \tag{3.4}$$

where a_i^l denotes the features of image i, $\tilde{N}_j$ denotes the number of images of examination j, and $\tilde{a}_j^l$ denotes the aggregated features.

For the problem of *where*, a CNN-based subnetwork is first used to extract features from the variable number of images in an examination. To reduce the parameters to learn, the first subnetwork is shared among the $\tilde{N}$ images in an examination. It has been proved that as the layers go deeper, higher-level features are extracted in CNNs. Some previous studies (He *et al.*, 2016a,b) have shown that deeper and wider networks contribute to better abstract ability of the CNNs. To explore the optimal abstract level to aggregate, different ls are tested. Based on the aggregated features, a second subnetwork is able to make the final prediction. The Inception-V2 network with feature aggregate operator in module 2 is presented in Fig. 3.6.

Training Method: CNNs with feature aggregate operators are trained with the backpropagation algorithm by minimizing the following cross-entropy cost function with respect to the parameters $\boldsymbol{\theta}$:

$$\mathcal{L} = -\frac{1}{M} \sum_{j=1}^{M} \boldsymbol{y}_j^\top \ln\left(\boldsymbol{a}_j^L\right), \tag{3.5}$$

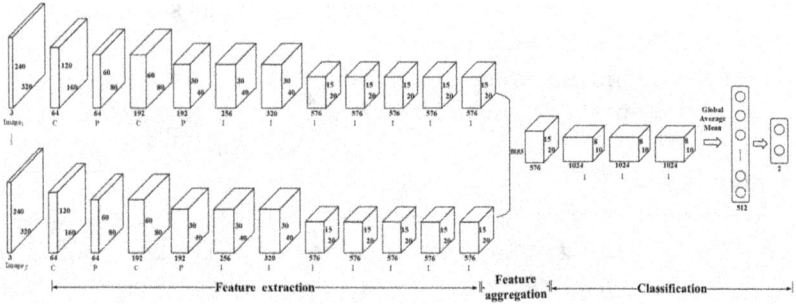

Fig. 3.6. Architecture of Inception-V2 with feature aggregate operator of max in module 2. The capital letters C, P, and I denote the Convolutional, Pooling, and Inception operations, respectively. The values represent the number of channels, widths, and heights of the feature maps.

where a^L denotes the output of the network after applying the softmax function. The cross-entropy cost function represents the similarities between the true distributions of labels and the approximated distributions of the network. The Adadelta algorithm (Zeiler, 2012) is used to minimizing the cost function. Different from the stochastic gradient descent (SGD) algorithm which has a fixed learning rate, Adadelta is an adaptive weight updates optimization method based on the first-order information. The Adadelta algorithm contains two parameters: one is the initial learning rate and the other is the decay rate used in the moving averages of the squared gradient.

3.4 Experimental Setup and Results

In this section, the experimental setup is presented, including the chosen evaluation strategy and implementation of the proposed method. The experimental results are then presented in detail.

3.4.1 *Experimental setup*

Configurations: The input of the model are RGB images in the size of $1600 \times 1200 \times 3$. To save computational resources, the original images are resized to $320 \times 240 \times 3$ with the OpenCV library (Bradski, 2000) through the bilinear interpolation. The resized images are then divided by 255, ensuring the pixel value is located between

0 and 1. The number of images per examination is set to 12. For the examination with the number of images less than 12, existing images are randomly chosen several times to round up to 12. Otherwise, 12 images are randomly selected from the examination. The parameters of the Adadelta optimizer are set according to the suggested values where the initial learning rate and the decay rate are 1.0 and 0.95, respectively. The weight updates are performed in mini-batches where the number of examinations per batch is 5. The training process is finished when up to 100 epochs.

Modern CNNs are typically constructed using blocks (e.g., Inception or Residual block) and divided into several modules. A module is composed of several blocks, and the feature maps in a module have identical sizes. To explore the effect of network architecture on the ROP recognition task, the VGG-16, Inception-V2, and ResNet-50 networks are tested. For VGG-16, the last two fully connected layers are replaced by the global average pooling (Lin *et al.*, 2013) which averages the feature maps along the spatial dimension to reduce overfitting. Table 3.3 shows the output size of each module in the networks. For each module in a specific network, the feature maps of the last block are aggregated.

Implementation: The proposed method is implemented using TensorFlow (Abadi *et al.*, 2016). All experiments are performed using a server with Linux OS and hardware of CPU Intel Xeon E5-2620@ 2.4GHz, GPU NVIDIA Tesla K40m, and 64 GB of RAM.

Table 3.3.   The output size of each module in VGG-16, Inception-V2, and ResNet-50 networks. The module in each network is stacked by blocks. The input images are down-sampled to 40 × 30 and 80 × 60 in the Inception-V2 and ResNet-50 respectively, through the max pooling and convolution with stride 2. Further details of the network architecture are provided in several previous studies (Simonyan and Zisserman, 2014; Ioffe and Szegedy, 2015; He *et al.*, 2016a).

Modules	VGG-16	Inception-V2	ResNet-50
Module 1	320 × 240	40 × 30	80 × 60
Module 2	160 × 120	20 × 15	40 × 30
Module 3	80 × 60	10 × 8	20 × 15
Module 4	40 × 30	\	10 × 8
Module 5	20 × 15	\	\

Evaluation Metrics: The training process is carried out on the training set, while the validation set is used to fine-tune the model. The overall performance of each model is assessed on the test set. Different metrics are calculated, including Accuracy, Sensitivity, Specificity, Precision, and F_1-score. The Receiver Operating Characteristic (ROC) and the Area Under Curve (AUC) are calculated to compare performances between models.

3.4.2 *Results*

(1) **Feature Aggregate Operators:** The performance of the proposed feature aggregate operators is described in the following. Table 3.4 shows the test accuracy of the proposed method for the classification of normal/ROP and mild/severe type of ROP. Performance between different networks is first compared. As seen in the table, Inception-V2 exhibits superior performance compared with VGG-16 and ResNet-50 in the two tasks. The high classification accuracy of Inception-V2 mainly benefited from the multiple operations in the Inception block (e.g., convolutional kernel size of 1×1, 3×3, and 5×5). These operations can extract variable features in multiple scales. For VGG-16 and ResNet-50, although the two CNNs

Table 3.4. Test accuracy of the proposed method in different network architectures for classification of normal/ROP and mild/severe ROP.

Networks	Modules	Normal and ROP		Mild and severe	
		Max	Mean	Max	Mean
VGG-16	Module 1	0.853	0.903	0.670	0.650
	Module 2	0.903	0.910	0.720	0.710
	Module 3	0.920	0.943	0.660	0.710
	Module 4	0.910	0.950	0.670	0.810
	Module 5	0.900	0.923	0.770	0.700
Inception-V2	Module 1	0.963	0.953	**0.840**	0.690
	Module 2	**0.970**	0.967	**0.840**	0.670
	Module 3	0.946	0.956	0.790	0.750
ResNet-50	Module 1	0.893	0.886	0.720	0.680
	Module 2	0.920	0.900	0.820	0.620
	Module 3	0.930	0.880	0.820	0.680
	Module 4	0.933	0.880	0.810	0.800

Note: The bold numbers highlight the better performance.

are designed to be deep enough to extract high-level features of the inputs, their performance oscillated more than that of Inception-V2 when aggregated in different modules. This is mainly caused by the fixed size of convolutional kernel (e.g., 3 × 3).

For the max and mean aggregation operators in Inception-V2, it can be seen from Table 3.4 that the max operator exhibits higher performance, except for module 3 in the classification of normal and ROP cases. Comparison of the performance of different modules in Inception-V2 in the classification of normal and ROP cases reveals the optimal feature for aggregation is in the middle of the network (e.g., module 2 with max aggregation operator yields the highest test accuracy of 0.97). Both modules 1 and 2 with the max aggregation operator achieved an accuracy of 0.84 in classifying mild and severe of ROP cases. It should be noted that test accuracy in the classification of normal and ROP is much higher than that of mild and severe ROP cases, indicating the latter task is substantially more difficult for the CNNs. This is consistent with the clinical diagnosis. Recognition of the severity of ROP is an intractable problem even for experienced ophthalmologists.

Figure 3.7 shows the training loss in Inception-V2 between the max and mean aggregation operators. The different aggregation modules in the max operator are also compared. Figures 3.7(a) and 3.7(b) show that the convergence speeds of module 1 and module 2 are higher than that of module 3 in the two classification tasks, suggesting that the classification subnetwork in is important for learning. Although the Inception-V2 with max aggregation operator in module 2 achieves the highest test accuracy of 0.97, greater oscillation can be observed after the 50th epoch. From Fig. 3.7(c), it can be seen that the convergence speed of the max operator is slightly higher than the mean in the classification of ROP and normal cases. The difference is magnified in the classification of mild and severe of ROP cases in Fig. 3.7(d), where the training loss of max aggregation declined rapidly compared with the mean.

(2) **Comparison With the State of the Art:** Table 3.5 shows a comparison of the proposed model with the first automated ROP detection system (Worrall *et al.*, 2016), which achieved better performance than traditional handcraft features. To implement the method proposed by Worrall *et al.*, a per-image classifier is established by assuming that the images in an examination shared the

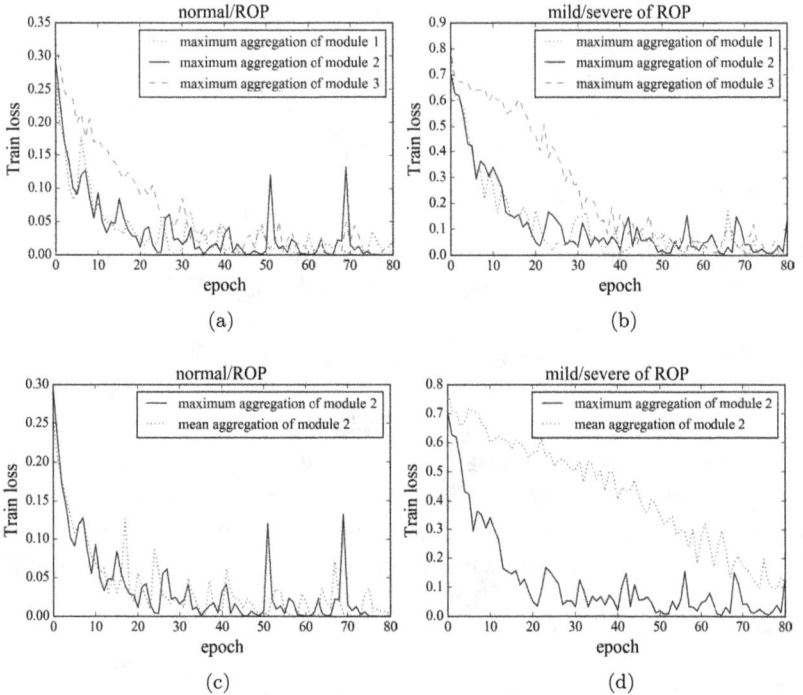

Fig. 3.7.   Comparison of training loss in Inception-V2 with different configurations. (a) training loss of Inception-V2 with max aggregation in the classification of normal and ROP cases, (b) training loss of Inception-V2 with max aggregation in the classification of mild and severe of ROP cases, (c) training loss of Inception-V2 with max and mean aggregation in the classification of normal and ROP cases, and (d) Training loss of Inception-V2 with max and mean aggregation in the classification of mild and severe of ROP cases.

Table 3.5.   Comparison of the proposed model with Worrall *et al.*' method

	Normal and ROP		Mild and Severe of ROP	
Metrics	Worrall *et al.*	Proposed	Worrall *et al.*	Proposed
Raw Acc	0.940	**0.970**	0.730	**0.840**
Sensitivity	0.926	**0.960**	**0.820**	**0.820**
Specificity	0.953	**0.980**	0.640	**0.860**
Precision	0.952	**0.979**	0.694	**0.854**
F1	0.939	**0.969**	0.752	**0.836**

Note: The bold numbers highlight the better performance.

same type of label. The classifier is based on an ImageNet pre-trained GoogLeNet and optimized by the RMSProp (Tieleman and Hinton, 2012) algorithm, as in Worrall *et al.*'s study. The model exhibiting the highest accuracy with the validation set is used in the per-examination classifier. For the classification of normal and ROP cases, the proposed model exhibited superior performance on all metrics. The test accuracy of the proposed model is 3% higher than that of Worrall *et al.*'s method, and the F1 score is also considerably higher. For the classification of mild and severe of ROP cases, the proposed model outperforms Worrall *et al.*'s method on most metrics except sensitivity, where the two models exhibit the same level of performance. The sensitivity and specificity of Worrall *et al.*'s method are 0.82 and 0.64, respectively, suggesting the model is preferable for predicting severe ROP. In the terms of F1 score, the performance of the proposed model is almost 11% higher than that of Worrall *et al.*'s method.

For a more detailed comparison at different operating points, ROC analysis is performed. Figure 3.8 shows the ROC curves and the AUC values for the proposed model and Worrall *et al.*'s method. In the classification of normal and ROP cases, the proposed model achieves superior performance. The ROC values of the proposed model and Worrall *et al.*'s method are 0.9922 and 0.9754, respectively. The superiority of the proposed model is more clearly observed in the classification of mild and severe of ROP cases, in which the AUC value of the proposed model is 15% higher than that in Worrall *et al.*'s method.

There are several possible explanations accounting for the superior performance of the proposed model compared with the method reported by Worrall *et al.*: (i) In the per-image classifier, Worrall *et al.* assumed that the images from an examination have the same type of label because the labels are based on the examination instead of the image. This assumption can't be fully verified because the images are taken from different views and with different artifacts. In some cases, it is difficult to determine whether an image exhibits disease-related characteristics or not from visual (e.g., 3.3(a)–3.3(c) and 3.3(e) in Fig. 3.3). (ii) In Worrall *et al.*'s model, recognition of ROP in an examination is based on the Beta distribution, which is determined by statistics based on the number of images classified as healthy and diseased in the training data. The parameters

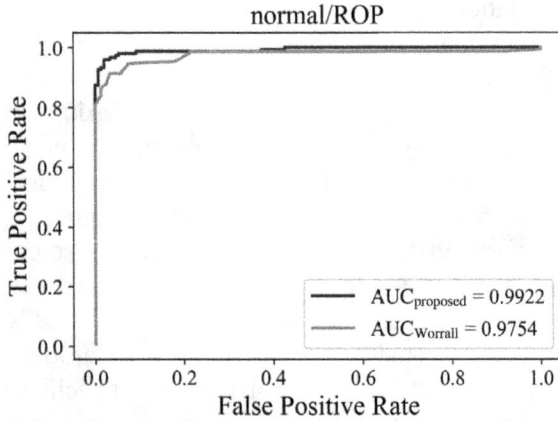

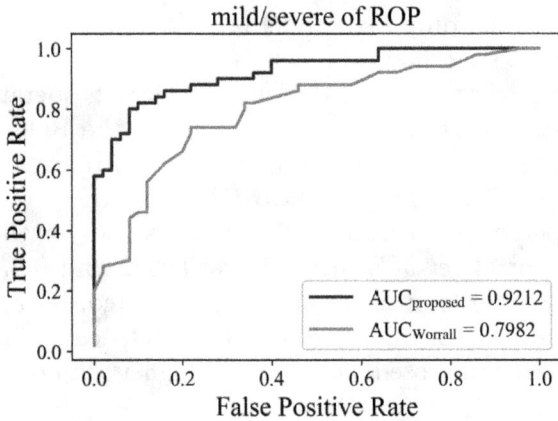

Fig. 3.8.   ROC analysis for the proposed model and Worrall *et al.*'s in the classification of normal/ROP and mild/severe of ROP.

of Beta distribution should be explicitly set up and can't be tuned by the gradient-based optimization method. In our work, the proposed model is trained to learn the disease-related characteristics from the data. Since the proposed method does not require prior knowledge about the distribution of the dataset, it may be more generalizable.

(3) **Visualization:** Visualization of the input images that most activate the softmax layer is presented in Fig. 3.9. The results are based

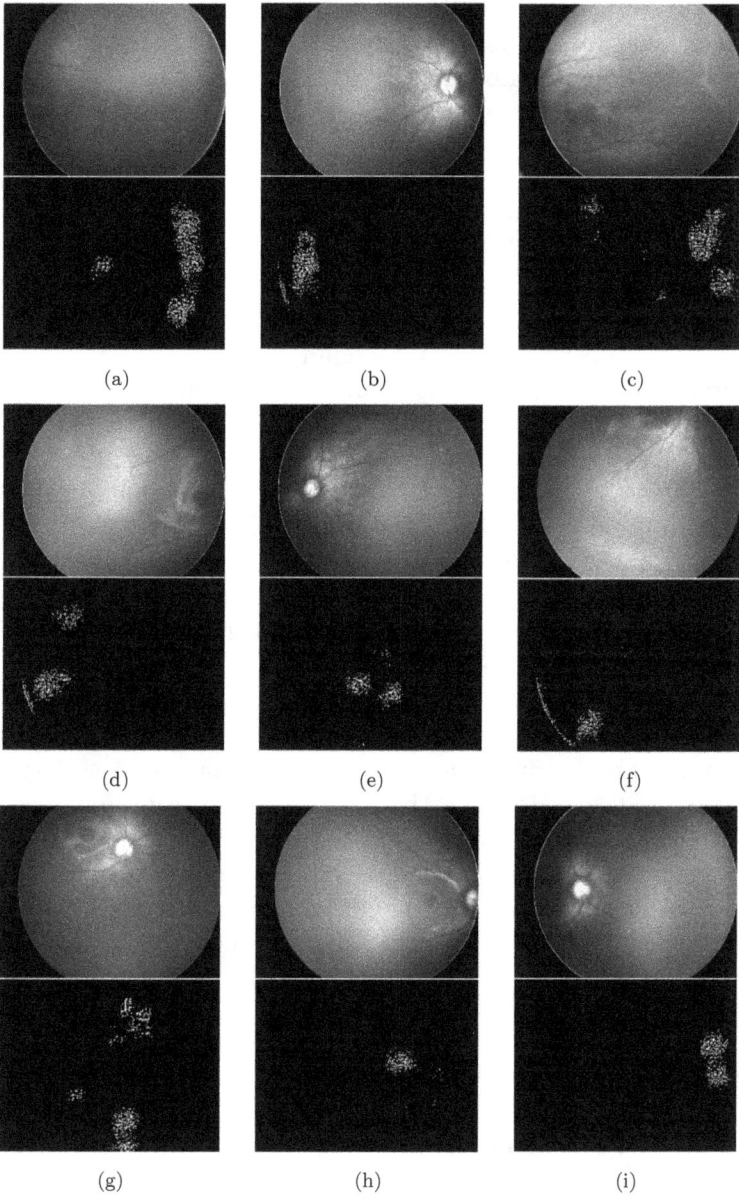

Fig. 3.9. Visualization of the input images in the test dataset that most activate the softmax layer with the guided backpropagation algorithm. The three
rows represent the images of the true positive, false negative, and false positive
examinations.

on the guided backpropagation algorithm (Springenberg *et al.*, 2014) in the classification of normal and ROP cases. The guided backpropagation algorithm computes the gradient of the activation of the specific neuron with regard to the inputs. The negative gradients which have inhibitory impact on the target neuron are masked out. Note that to improve the visualization performance, the generated gradient images are binarized. The images in the first row are from true positive examinations. By comparing the input images with the corresponding visualization results, it is clear that the output of the softmax layer is highly correlated with the ridge area in the input images. This is consistent with the guidelines for clinicians, in which the ridge in the fundus is important for the diagnosis of ROP. The visualization results demonstrate that the proposed model learned to extract the essential features for the diagnosis of ROP, despite the shapes and orientations of the ridge. For example, the model recognized the ridge in Figs. 3.9(a) and 3.9(b), located at the left and right parts of the images, respectively. Even when the ridge has a different shape, the model is still able to recognize it (e.g., Fig. 3.9(c)).

The second row in Fig. 3.9 shows images from a false negative examination. Figure 3.9(d) shows that the ridge located in the top-left part of the image is successfully identified, along with the down-left area which has no obvious disease-related features from the visual. The fundus image in Fig. 3.9(f) shows apparent ROP-indicative features. However, the model failed to accurately recognize all the lesions but only the left part of it. The images that belong to a false positive examination can be seen at the third row in Fig. 3.9. As shown in Fig. 3.9(g), the model associates the prediction result with the optic disc and the lower area in the fundus image. From Figs. 3.9(h) and 3.9(i), it can be seen that the model falsely recognizes the reflection of light as the ridge of ROP, leading to an incorrect prediction result.

(4) **Analytic Experiments:** In this subsection, two experiments are performed to validate the proposed model. One is to test the impact of the number of ROP-related images on the model, and the other is to examine the model's classification performance of examinations from premature infants.

The model's performance change according to the number of ROP-related images in test dataset is illustrated in Table 3.6. The

Table 3.6.   Statistics of the number of ROP-related images in test dataset.

Number of ROP-related images	1	2	3	4	5	6	≥ 7
Number of examinations annotated as ROP	35	38	20	24	10	12	11
Number of wrong predicted examinations	2	3	0	1	0	0	0

second row in Table 3.6 represents the number of examinations annotated as ROP case. The third row represents the number of misclassified examinations. It can be seen from the table that there are two and three examinations with one and two ROP-related images misclassified, respectively. The model misclassified one examination with four ROP-related images. Examinations with more than five ROP-related images are all correctly predicted as ROP.

To further validate the proposed model, 406 examinations collected in January 2018 from 195 premature infants (birth weight ≤ 2500 grams or gestational age ≤ 28 weeks) are used as test dataset after the annotation phases. The data annotation phases are kept the same as described in Section 2.3. These premature infants have not appeared in the dataset used to construct the model. Figures 3.10(a) and 3.10(b) show the confusion matrix of the normal/ROP and mild/severe ROP classification tasks, respectively. It can be seen from Fig. 3.10(a) that the model accurately recognized most normal examinations (352 out of 356) but misclassified five ROP examinations. This is mainly due to the diversity of the characteristics of ROP. In the classification of mild/severe of ROP, the model only misclassified one examination in each class. The results further demonstrate the effectiveness of the proposed model in diagnosing ROP.

3.5   Clinical Application of DeepROP

Clinically speaking, the diagnosis of ROP involves two departments: neonatology and ophthalmology. Figure 3.11 illustrates the process of diagnosis in a hospital. The premature infant is generally observed in the neonatology department, and the neonatologist will use a range of professional equipment, such as RetCAM, to evaluate the infant's

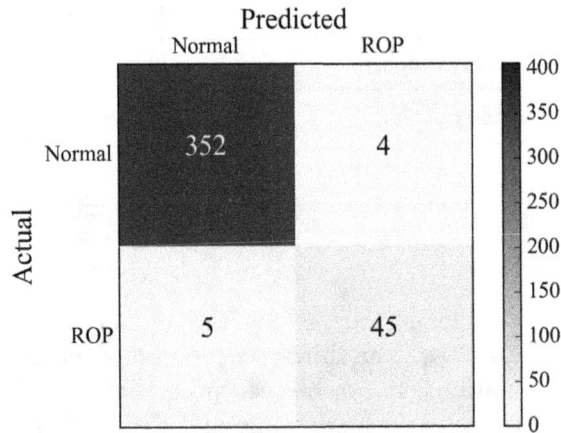

(a)

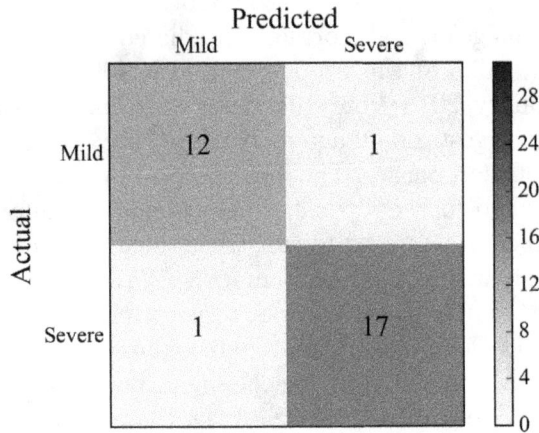

(b)

Fig. 3.10.   The confusion matrix of the two classification tasks. (a) and (b) Represent the normal/ROP and mild/severe of ROP classification tasks, respectively.

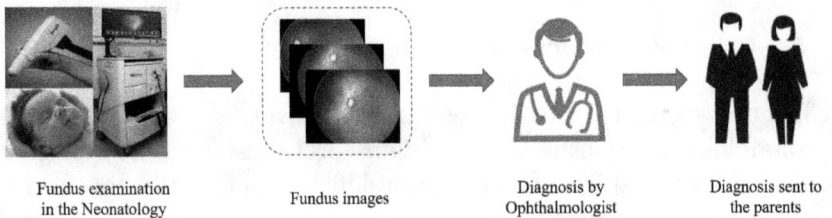

Fundus examination   Fundus images   Diagnosis by   Diagnosis sent to
in the Neonatology   Ophthalmologist   the parents

Fig. 3.11.   Workflow of the traditional fundus examination.

fundus development. The ophthalmologist then diagnoses the collected fundus photographs, after which he/she notifies the doctors in the neonatology department and the baby's parents of the results. Since the whole process involves the interaction between the two departments of neonatology and ophthalmology, the whole process (from the initial neonatal fundus examination to the parents finally learning the diagnosis results) takes 3–5 days, which may delay the timely treatment of children with serious fundus diseases. In view of these pain points, we constructed an intelligent-aided diagnosis system for retinopathy of prematurity, called DeepROP, which aims to accurately identify the lesion and accelerate the process of lesion diagnosis using the deep neural network model constructed above. The system participated in the 2019 "National College Artificial Intelligence Innovation Competition" and stood out from more than 200 teams across the country, ultimately winning first prize. This section will introduce the system framework, system implementation, and clinical application.

3.5.1 *System framework*

DeepROP comprises two parts, namely the system terminal for neonatology and the smartphone terminal for ophthalmologists and parents. The overall workflow of the system is illustrated in Fig. 3.12. For a new examination case, after the neonatologist has completed the fundus examination, the system will monitor the locally generated fundus examination data and automatically upload the data of the case to the cloud server, as shown in Step 2 in Fig. 3.12. After the server receives the data, it stores the fundus photo in the database in the form of image files, along with information related to the infant (such as the infant's ID, gestational age, and weight).

The deep neural network model is constructed to identify the existence and severity of lesions, as shown in Step 3 in Fig. 3.12. After obtaining the results predicted by the model, the system will automatically push the results to the ophthalmologist's smartphone via WeChat, notifying the doctor that there is a new case to be viewed.

The ophthalmologist can make a decision by viewing the fundus photos and the AI prediction results. After the fifth step of the doctor's review is complete, the system will push the diagnosis completion message to the parents's smartphone via WeChat; subsequently,

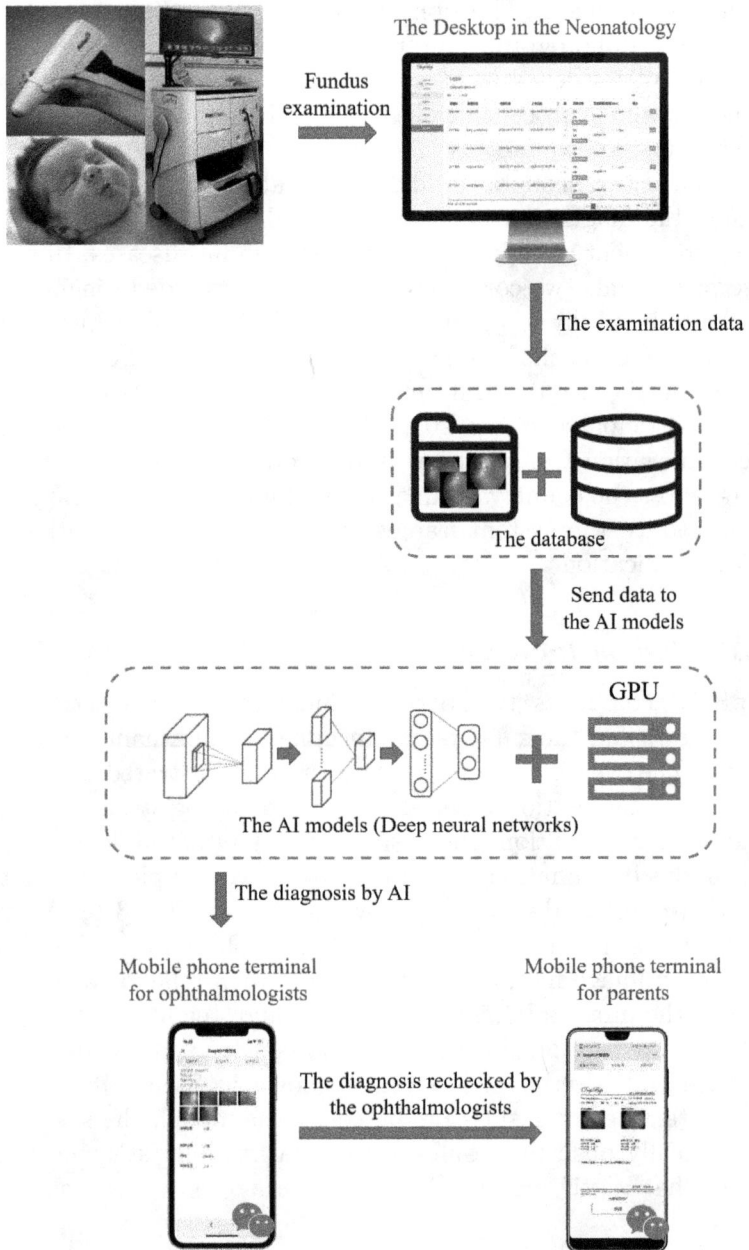

Fundus examination

The Desktop in the Neonatology

The examination data

The database

Send data to the AI models

GPU

The AI models (Deep neural networks)

The diagnosis by AI

Mobile phone terminal for ophthalmologists

Mobile phone terminal for parents

The diagnosis rechecked by the ophthalmologists

Fig. 3.12. Workflow of the DeepROP.

parents can directly view the fundus photos and the results of the doctor's diagnosis.

As can be seen from the above workflow, the system automatically uploads the underlying data, predicts the results, and pushes messages. Practical applications have shown that the system shortens the average time required to diagnose the lesion from three to five days to several minutes, which greatly expedites the diagnosis process performed by ophthalmologists.

The DeepROP contains three main modules: the data management module, AI module, and user management module. Here, the main functions of the data management module are automatic data uploading, data storage, data retrieval, and data statistics. The AI module mainly uses a trained deep neural network model to provide predictive services. For its part, the user management module incorporates user login and user information maintenance functions.

The mobile phone terminal is divided into three parts, namely the doctor's terminal, the parent's terminal, and the message push module. Of these, the doctor's terminal contains functions that facilitate user login, viewing the fundus photos, and transmitting the diagnostic results. The functions of the parents terminal are similar to those of the doctor's terminal, except that the review and diagnosis function is replaced by a diagnostic report viewing function. The message push module is responsible for the message push of the mobile phone terminal, which realizes the push of the doctor's terminal to be reviewed, and the diagnostic message push function of the parents terminal.

3.5.2 *System implementation*

DeepROP was released in September 2017 in the Neonatology Department of Chengdu Women and Children's Center Hospital. From its release until March in 2020, it served a total of 15,725 person-times, effectively improving the work efficiency of neonatology and ophthalmologists. This subsection will introduce the specific implementation of the neonatology system, the doctor's mobile phone terminal, and the parents' mobile phone terminal.

(1) **Desktop in the neonatology department:** The system is a B/S architecture; in addition to the cloud server, there is also a data

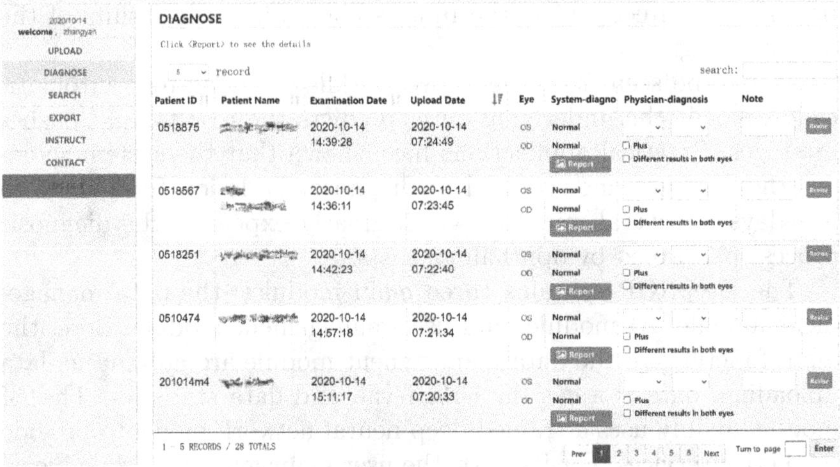

Fig. 3.13.   Data browsing in the desktop in the neonatology department.

monitoring service deployed in the neonatology department, which is used to obtain the fundus data of the newly examined eye in real time and automatically upload it to the cloud server. Figure 3.13 presents the "Today's Diagnostics" page in the system, which lists all fundus examination data for the day and gives the identification results generated by the AI model.

In order to facilitate data management, the system supports a variety of search methods, including searching by the infant's ID, the infant's name, the date of data upload, and the date of examination. Figure 3.14 lists the data retrieved between May 1st, 2020 and May 30th, 2020 for partial searches. In addition, the system also supports the exporting of historical diagnostic records in Excel format, which enables the doctor to summarize the data.

(2) **Doctor's Mobile Phone Terminal:** After the device in the neonatology department has automatically uploaded the data to the server and the recognition result has been generated by the AI model, the doctor's mobile phone terminal receives a notification from the system, as shown in Fig. 3.15(a). By clicking on the notification message, the doctor will enter the main interface of the doctor's mobile phone terminal, as shown in Fig. 3.15(b). The bottom of the page contains three columns, labeled "to be diagnosed", "to be reviewed", and "diagnosed", which correspond to the three states of the infant's

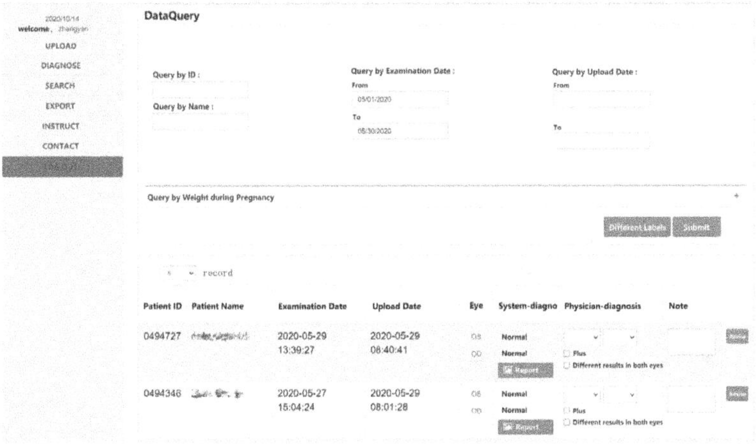

Fig. 3.14. Data retrieval in the desktop in the neonatology department.

diagnosis. The "Pending Diagnosis" list corresponds to cases that have been accepted by the doctor but have not yet been diagnosed; "Pending Review" lists cases in which the doctor is unsure of the medical condition, which are assigned a pending state while awaiting further confirmation; finally, "Diagnosed" contains those cases for which a doctor has provided a diagnosis.

By clicking the appropriate button (as shown in Fig. 3.15(b)), the doctor can view the fundus images of an individual case (as shown in Fig. 3.15(c)). The interface is divided into left/right eye to show the infant's fundus images, the diagnosis results of the AI model. The ophthalmologist can also recheck the stage of the ROP, region of the ROP, and plus existence, as well as view a specific image in a larger full-screen format by clicking on the fundus thumbnail. Furthermore, the ophthalmologist can also select the representative fundus image that will be displayed in the diagnostic report received by the parent. After diagnosing the infant's left/right eye, the ophthalmologist can fill in specific medical advice information in the diagnostic opinion page, as shown in Fig. 3.15(d).

(3) **Parents' Mobile Phone Terminal:** The parents have to bind their WeChat ID to their babies when registered in the system (as shown in Fig. 3.16(a)). After the ophthalmologist completes the diagnosis of the infant via his/her mobile phone, the parent's terminal will receive a notification from the system (as shown in Fig. 3.16(b)).

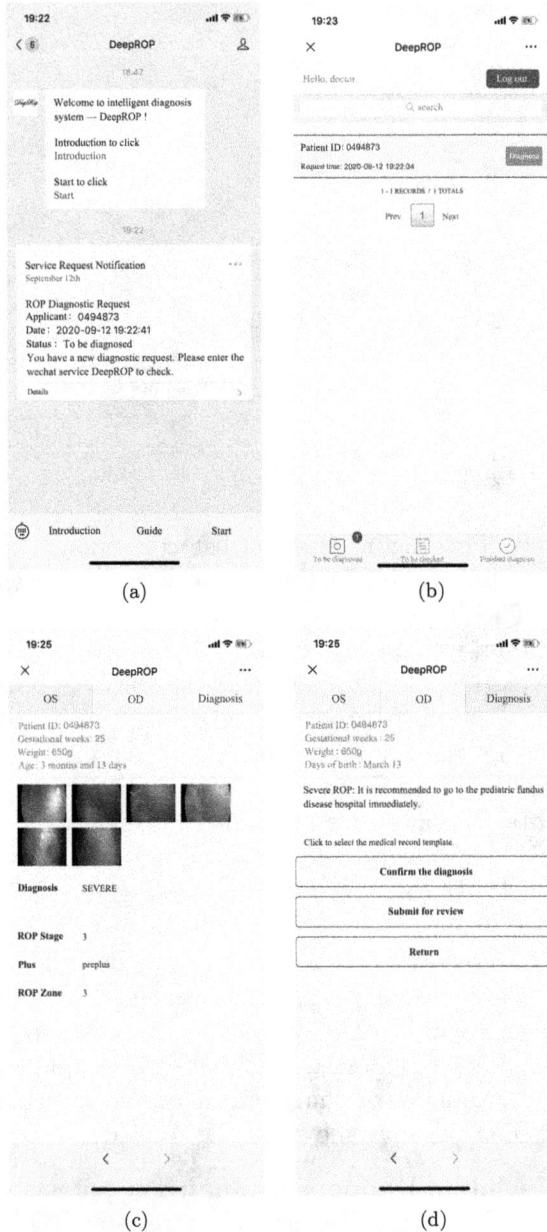

Fig. 3.15.   The Doctor's mobile phone terminal.

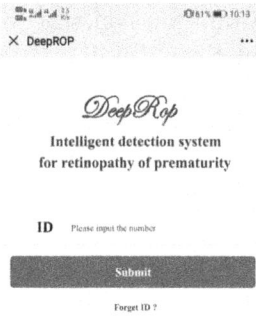

(a)

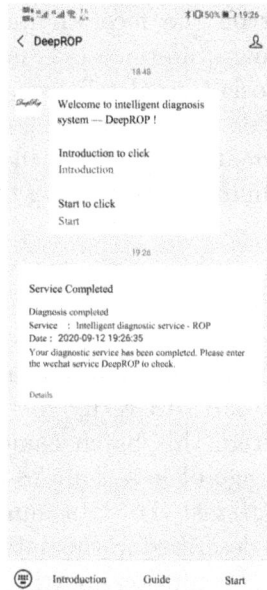

(b)

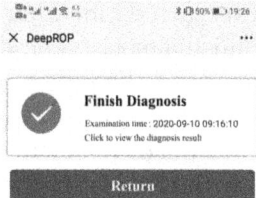

(c)

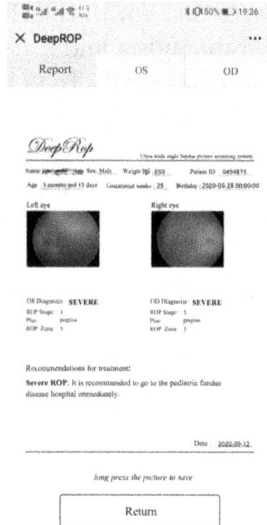

(d)

Fig. 3.16.   The Parents's mobile phone terminal.

By clicking on the received message notification, the parents will enter the main interface (as shown in Fig. 3.16(c)). By clicking on the "Diagnosis Complete" area, they can view the diagnostic report that has been automatically generated based on the doctor's diagnostic information (as shown in Fig. 3.16(d)) and switch to view the left/right fundus images using the Tab bar.

3.5.3   *Clinical application*

After DeepROP was released, we collected and annotated 406 examination data from Chengdu Women and Children's Central Hospital in February 2018 to verify the practical application of the system. The data from this batch came from 195 infants with an average gestational age of less than 28 and an average birth weight of less than 2500 grams; the data annotation process was consistent with the process described in the data preparation subsection. Figure 4.14 presents the confusion matrix for this batch of data predictions. For ROP recognition tasks, the system successfully identified 352 of the 356 cases of normal fundus examination, in addition to five cases that were missed. In the ROP severity identification task, there was 1 missed diagnosis and 1 case of misdiagnosis. These identification results further verify the effectiveness of the model proposed in this paper.

DeepROP was developed based on the needs of clinical practical application. It operates in accordance with the workflow of neonatology and ophthalmologists to the greatest extent possible and assists doctors with completing the diagnosis of lesions. Notably, the model's identification results need to be reviewed and confirmed by the ophthalmologist, who will provide a diagnostic opinion before the results are pushed to the parent's WeChat terminal; this will ensure that missed diagnosis and misdiagnosis are minimized to the greatest possible extent.

3.6   Conclusion

In this chapter, a novel architecture of CNNs is proposed to recognize the existence and severity of ROP. The architecture is composed of a feature extract subnetwork, followed by a feature aggregate operator to bind features from variable images in an examination. The prediction is accomplished using a second subnetwork with the aggregated features as inputs. Max and mean aggregate operators are explored based on the architecture. Several ImageNet pretrained networks are tested in the study, including VGG-16, Inception-V2, and ResNet50. The proposed architecture is verified with a large dataset of 2668 examinations of the fundus in infants. The experimental results demonstrate that the Inception-V2 with the max aggregate operator in module 2 is a proper network architecture for the recognition of the existence and severity of ROP. Compared with the mean aggregate operator, the max has better classification accuracy and convergence speed. Meanwhile, a patient's multiple examinations in train, validation, and test datasets have little impact on model's performance, mainly because the characteristics of the eyes of the premature infants are varied over time.

The visualization results demonstrate that the proposed architecture learned the clinical characteristics of ROP, despite the location and shape of the ridge in ROP. However, the reflection of light in the image may impact the recognition result of the model. The proposed model also outperformed the state of the art, verifying the effectiveness of our proposed architecture. In future studies, we will extend the method to diagnose the plus disease in ROP and integrate the recognition of stage and plus disease to aid ophthalmologists in clinical diagnosis.

Based on the trained ROP recognition model, we further construct an intelligent auxiliary diagnosis system, named DeepROP, which is composed of a system terminal deployed in the neonatology department and mobile phone terminals for ophthalmologists and parents. The system has been applied in Chengdu Women and Children's Central Hospital and has completed a total of 15,725 service trips. Findings show that the proposed DeepROP effectively reduces the workload of doctors, accelerates the process of diagnosing children, and has been unanimously recognized by doctors in practical applications.

Chapter 4

Diagnosis of Diabetic Retinopathy Using Deep Neural Networks

Diabetic retinopathy (DR) is a common eye disease and a significant cause of blindness in diabetic patients. Regular screening with fundus photography and timely intervention is the most effective way to manage the disease. The large population of diabetic patients and their massive screening requirements have generated interest in computer-aided and fully automatic diagnosis of DR. Deep neural networks, on the other hand, have brought many breakthroughs in various tasks in recent years. To automate the diagnosis of DR and provide the appropriate suggestions to DR patients, we have built a dataset of DR fundus images that have been labeled by the proper treatment method that is required. Using this dataset, we trained deep convolutional neural network models to grade the severities of DR fundus images. We were able to achieve an accuracy of 88.72% for a four-degree classification task in the experiments. We deployed our models on a cloud computing platform and provided pilot DR diagnostic services for several hospitals, in the clinical evaluation the system achieved a consistency rate of 91.8% with ophthalmologists, demonstrating the effectiveness of our work.

4.1   Introduction

Diabetic retinopathy (DR) is the most common cause of blindness among diabetic patients (Fong *et al.*, 2004). According to the World

Health Organization (WHO), there were 422 million diabetic patients in 2014, 35% of whom developed some type of retinopathy owing to the accumulation of damage to small blood vessels in the retina (World Health Organization, 2016). The prevalence of DR is much higher among special groups of patients. For example, it is estimated that 40% of type II diabetic patients and 86% of type I diabetic patients in the US have DR, and the rate of DR is estimated to be 43% in rural areas of China (Ning Cheung, 2010).

The loss of sight can vary during the gradual development of DR. Generally, DR can be separated into two major stages: nonproliferative DR (NPDR) and proliferative DR (PDR), which is characterized by neovascularization or vitreous/preretinal hemorrhage. Up to 10% of diabetic patients who have no DR will develop NPDR annually, and for patients with severe NPDR, the risk of developing PDR in one year is 75%. The shift from normal status (no apparent abnormality in the retina) to PDR commonly takes many years. Thus, NPDR is often divided into three substages: mild, moderate, and severe NPDR. Together, these five stages make up the widely used "International Clinical Diabetic Retinopathy Disease Severity Scale" (Ophthalmoscopy and Levels, 2002). The best treatment options for patients differ between stages. For patients with no DR or mild NPDR, only regular screening is required; for patients with moderate NPDR or worse, the treatment options vary from scatter laser treatment to vitrectomy. Thus, to provide patients with the appropriate treatment, it is important to first grade their DR severity. Clinically, the diagnosis of DR is often made with fundus images, which can be acquired by photographing the fundus directly. The common lesions that indicate DR include hard or soft exudates, microaneurysms, and hemorrhages. All of these lesions can be identified from fundus images; Figure 4.1 shows sample fundus images containing various types of lesions. To make a more accurate diagnosis, fluorescein angiography can be used because it can reveal fine vessel structures in the retina. However, fluorescein dyes can cause an allergic reaction and require functioning kidneys to excrete, and they are usually not available in small hospitals. Currently, fundus images are the most widely used approach for regular screening of DR, since the acquisition of such images is convenient and the visibility of most lesions is sufficient.

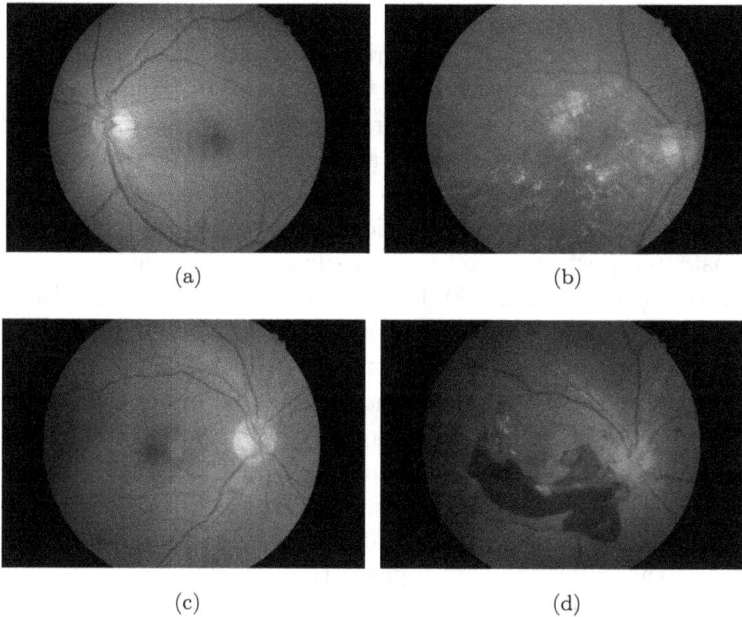

Fig. 4.1. Sample fundus images with different types of lesions. (a) A normal fundus, (b) fundus with exudates, (c) fundus with microaneurysms, and (d) fundus with hemorrhages.

Although the equipment for fundus photography can be accessed easily, a qualified ophthalmologist who can analyze the fundus images cannot. The population of diabetic patients is enormous, and the prevalence of diabetes has been rising rapidly — the global prevalence of diabetes among adults has increased from 4.7% in 1980 to 8.5% in 2014 (World Health Organization, 2016). Yet, experienced ophthalmologists are rare and are distributed unevenly; the total number of ophthalmologists worldwide in 2012 was 210,730 (i.e., 29 ophthalmologists per 1 million persons) (Resnikoff *et al.*, 2012). For middle- and low-income countries, the gap between the population of diabetic patients and ophthalmologists can be extremely wide, indicating an urgent need for systems that diagnose DR automatically.

Much work has been done in using computers to make automatic DR diagnoses. Traditional methods often deploy various feature extraction modules to first extract useful information from fundus images. Then, the extracted features are fed into certain classifiers, such as random forest, support vector machine, and the AdaBoost classifier. Such hand-crafted feature-based methods are laborious and often fail to yield good results.

In the recent decade, deep neural networks (DNNs) have achieved revolutionary results in many areas. They bring about break-throughs in computer vision, speech recognition, and natural language processing. Many applications of deep neural networks have demonstrated performance that can surpass human beings, e.g., face recognition (Sun *et al.*, 2015), large-scale visual recognition (He *et al.*, 2015a), and the game of Go (Silver *et al.*, 2016). The use of DNNs in the diagnosis of DR has also attracted much interest, and much progress has been made. However, despite the many advances that have been made, clinical application of automatic DR diagnosis systems remains unavailable and many works still need to be done.

In this paper, we propose a new dataset of fundus images for grading DR. In contrast to existing scales that grade fundus images mainly by the pathological changes in the retina, we take into account clinical practice, i.e., we grade a fundus image based on its abnormalities and required treatment method. For example, patients with severe NPDR and mild PDR are recommended to undergo laser scatter treatment; thus, we group them in the same category. With this dataset, several deep convolutional neural network (DCNN) models were trained for the diagnosis of DR. We also propose a new model which is better adapted to small lesions in the fundus images. The experimental results show that our work achieves state-of-the-art performance compared with other works on similar tasks. Our models were also deployed for clinical evaluation in several hospitals, performing nearly as well as ophthalmologists.

4.2 Related Works

In the decades-long seeking for automatic DR diagnosis, many works have been done. We summarize related works briefly from three aspects. First, we list the most related datasets that are constructed for DR-related tasks. Second, we summarize related works using traditional image processing techniques. In the end, we showcase some recent works that use various convolutional neural network (CNN) models.

4.2.1   Related dataset

Various datasets of fundus images for DR-related diagnoses have been developed, including the following:

- Standard Diabetic Retinopathy Database Calibration Level 0/1 (DIARETDB0/DIARETDB1) dataset (Kauppi *et al.*, 2006, 2007),
- Methods to Evaluate Segmentation and Indexing techniques in the field of Retinal Ophthalmology (MESSIDOR) dataset (Decencière *et al.*, 2014),
- Digital Retinal Images for Vessel Extraction (DRIVE) dataset (Staal *et al.*, 2004),
- STructured Analysis of the Retina (STARE) dataset (Hoover *et al.*, 2000),
- Retinal Vessel Image set for Estimation of Widths (REVIEW) dataset (Al-Diri *et al.*, 2008),
- Kaggle Diabetic Retinopathy dataset (Kaggle, 2016),
- E-ophtha dataset (Decencière *et al.*, 2013).

These datasets differ significantly in their annotation, for that they were proposed for different tasks. For example, in the DIARETDB0 dataset, the type and position of each abnormality are labeled in detail, whereas in the Kaggle DR dataset, the label for each image is a simple integer indicating one of five degrees of severity. The sizes of these datasets also differ. The REVIEW dataset contains only 16 images, and the DIARETDB0 dataset contains 130 images, while the Kaggle dataset contains up to 88,702 images. Further, the quality of the annotations varies significantly.

4.2.2   Traditional practice

Traditional image classification pipelines can be divided roughly into three main stages: image preprocessing, feature extraction, and feature classification. For the diagnosis of DR, there are studies for each of these stages. For example, Rubini *et al.* proposed to apply hessian-based candidate selection before the feature extraction and classification using a support vector machine (SVM) classifier (Rubini and Kunthavai, 2015). Mookiah *et al.* proposed a system that used hybrid features, including exudate/vessel area, texture, and entropy, for DR classification (Mookiah *et al.*, 2013). Bhatkar *et al.* explored the use of the multi-layer perception neural network as the classifier to process extracted features, such as a 64-point discrete cosine transform, and other statistical features, including entropy and Euler's number (Bhatkar and Kharat, 2015).

Despite the performance of these approaches, the drawbacks of traditional methods are obvious. On one hand, given that simple and direct features are already exploited, crafting new effective features by hand becomes more difficult. On the other hand, the performance of these approaches plateaus, which makes them harder to improve.

4.2.3   *Deep convolutional neural network approaches*

Deep neural networks, especially convolutional ones, have demonstrated their superiority in image classification tasks. Many CNN-based methods have been introduced for making automatic DR diagnoses. For example, Gulshan *et al.* proposed to use the Inception-V3 as their architecture for detecting DR (Gulshan *et al.*, 2016). Quellec *et al.* created heatmaps of the image to show the role of each pixel for classification and used a generalization of backpropagation for training CNNs to create the heatmaps (Quellec *et al.*, 2017). Yang *et al.* proposed a two-stage DCNN-based algorithm that detects lesions in fundus images and grades the severity of DR (Yang *et al.*, 2017). Chandore *et al.* trained a DCNN model on a large dataset to detect the symptoms of DR from fundus images (Chandore and Asati, 2017).

Although much progress has been made with these CNN-based approaches, there are still gaps between the current results and their clinical application. First of all, many works were done on subtasks of the problem, such as vessel segmentation or detecting lesions of specific kinds. Second, many experimental results were achieved on very small datasets and thus lack persuasion for real-world applications. For example, the accuracies for vessel segmentation on the DRIVE and STARE datasets can be achieved as 97.67% and 98.13% (Wang *et al.*, 2015), however vessel segmentation alone cannot be used as diagnosis of DR. The accuracies for lesion detection on the DIARETDB0 and DIARETDB1 datasets can be achieved as 96.0% and 94.6% (Adarsh and Jeyakumari, 2013), however the presence of certain lesions can only be used as supporting evidence and the diagnosis is up to ophthalmologists who use these facts. It should also be noted that for these subtasks, the size of datasets is often small, i.e., the number of total images in the STARE, DRIVE, DIARETDB0, and DIARETDB1 datasets are only 20, 40, 130, and 89, respectively. For the DR severity grading task, performance of previous works is relatively low, for example, in (Chandore and Asati, 2017), only two classes were considered (with and without DR), and the accuracies for the two classes were not practical (with DR 0.88 and without DR 0.81). In (Yang *et al.*, 2017), the accuracy for the four grades of NPDR was less than 60%, and the accuracy for another subset of the Kaggle dataset was 75% (Pratt *et al.*, 2016).

4.3   Overview

Our aim was to build a model that can grade the severity of DR in a given fundus image. To this end, we performed the following steps, as shown in Figure 4.2:

(1) data collection,
(2) data annotation,
(3) data preprocessing,
(4) data augmentation,
(5) model setup and evaluation,
(6) model deployment,
(7) clinical evaluation.

To describe these steps in detail, the rest of this chapter is organized into five sections. In the dataset construction section, we describe how our data were collected and annotated and provide a detailed annotation scheme and our rationale for such a scheme. In the data preprocessing and augmentation section, the preprocessing pipeline for unifying images from different sources is described. The augmentation techniques in our work are also introduced in this section. In the model section, basic ideas and computational principles of DCNNs are described. Then, the models we use are described. In the experiments section, detailed descriptions for various experiments are included, and the experiment results are discussed and analyzed using visualization techniques. To evaluate our work in real clinical

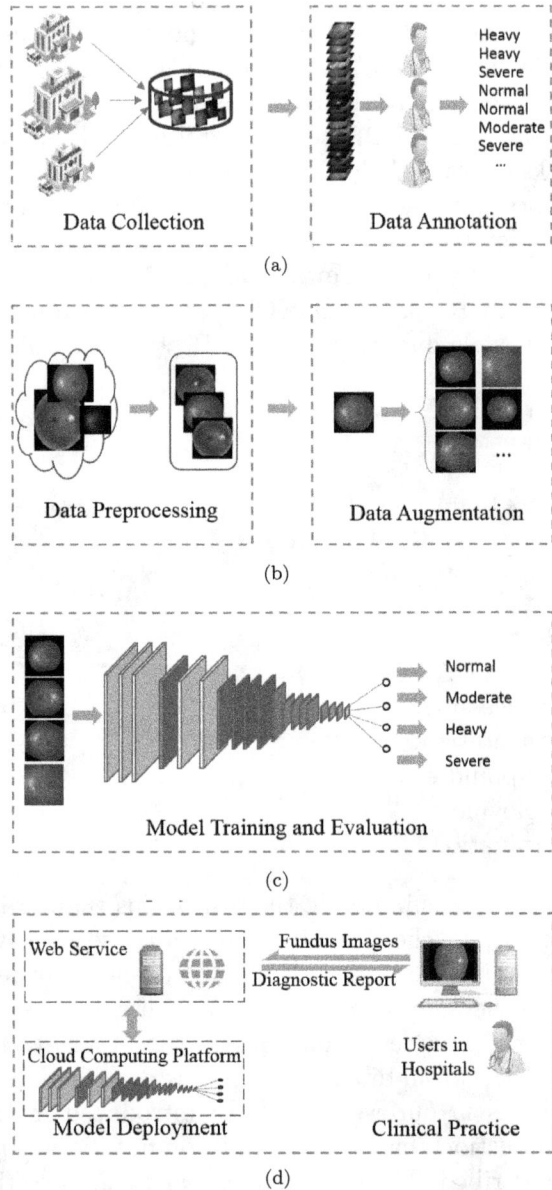

Fig. 4.2. The framework of this work. (a) Dataset construction, (b) data preparation, (c) DR diagnosis with DCNN, and (d) model deployment and clinical practice.

environments, we deploy our models on a cloud computing platform and provide a pilot diagnostic service to several hospitals in nearby cities. These works are introduced in the model deployment and clinical evaluation section. Finally, we present the conclusion section.

4.4   Dataset Construction

In addition to the existing datasets mentioned above, we have constructed a novel dataset of fundus images. Each image in the dataset is labeled with one of the four degrees of DR severity. Our dataset is moderate in size, totaling 4476 images from three clinical departments (the Ophthalmology Department, Health Management Center, and Endocrinology & Metabolism Department) at Sichuan Provincial People's Hospital, which ranks second in Ophthalmology in Sichuan Province. After the data collection, three senior ophthalmologists were invited to label each of these images. Each image is labeled by them independently; for images labeled with inconsistency, discussions were held to achieve a final result. For patients from the Ophthalmology Department, the original diagnosis reports with fluorescein angiography were also used to facilitate the discussions. The fundus images in our dataset were labeled with one of the four degrees: Normal, Moderate, Heavy, and Severe. The relationship between these degrees and those degrees in Ophthalmoscopy and Levels (2002) is listed in Table 4.1, as are the corresponding treatment suggestions for each degree. The annotation criteria that we used differed slightly from that of other datasets. There are two major reasons for this choice. The first is that, for ophthalmologists, the progression from severe NPDR to mild PDR is sometimes obscure or even unrecognizable from fundus images. If necessary, a fluorescein angiography is proper for a more precise diagnosis. The second is that the suggested treatments are same for mild and moderate NPDR patients or severe NPDR and mild PDR patients. Thus, it is convenient to group them together for clinical practice. In Fig. 4.3, we show sample images with the corresponding labels from our annotation.

Table 4.1. The annotation scheme in this work.

Severity level	Observable findings on fundus images	Corresponding category in Ophthalmoscopy and Levels (2002)	Suggested treatment
Normal	No abnormalities	Normal	Recheck in 12 months
Moderate	Microaneurysm, exudation, but less than Heavy	Mild or moderate NPDR	Recheck in 6 months
Heavy	Any of the following: 1. More than 20 intraretinal hemorrhages in each of the 4 quadrants 2. Definite venous beading in 2+ quadrants 3. Prominent IRMA in 1+ quadrant 4. PDR but less than severe	Severe NPDR or mild PDR	Scatter laser treatment
Severe	One or more of the following: Premacular hemorrhage, vitreous hemorrhage, severe retinal proliferative	Severe PDR	Laser or vitrectomy treatment

4.5 Data Preprocessing and Augmentation

4.5.1 *Preprocessing*

One problem that we face is the variety of fundus image capture devices; because the techniques that are required for the manufacture of such devices are mature and open, various companies have developed dozens of such products, each of which generates fundus images to a particular standard. To ensure that machines learn the true features of DR rather than device-specific information, we need to process the acquired fundus images from different sources and change them into a uniform format through the following steps:

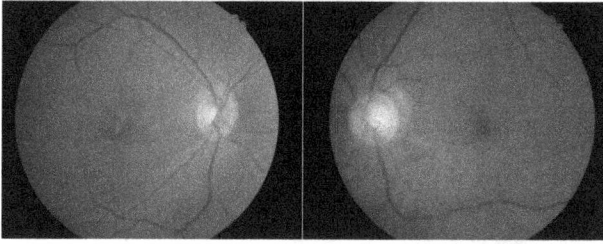

(a)

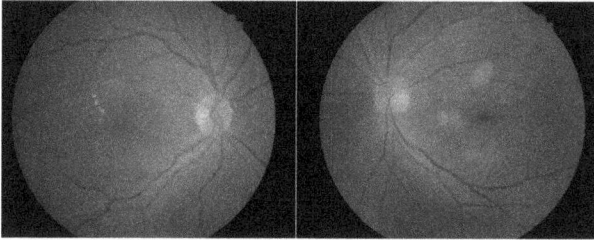

(b)

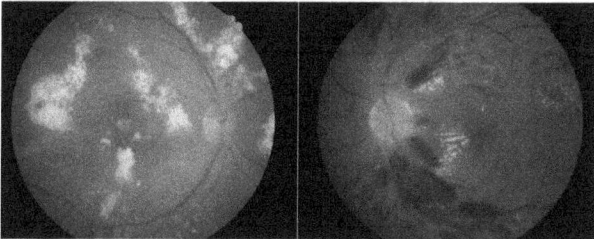

(c)

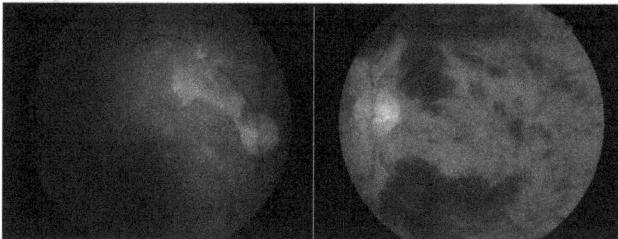

(d)

Fig. 4.3. Sample fundus images and corresponding labels. (a) Normal, (b) moderate, (c) heavy, and (d) severe.

4.5.1.1   *Size normalization*

The first step is to resize different images into a uniform scale so that all fundus areas in different images have the same diameter. The black borders on each side of the fundus image are removed at the outset by summing the images horizontally and vertically and discarding regions that correspond to values under a selected threshold. Then, the images are resized to fixed dimensions.

4.5.1.2   *Shape normalization*

Some fundus images are complete circles, whereas others may lack the top and bottom margins. In addition, many devices capture a small notch on the edge of the circle. To unify the shapes of these images, we use a mask that contains the largest common area of all images from different sources to obscure unwanted parts of the image.

4.5.1.3   *Color normalization*

After the shape of each image is normalized, its color must be tuned because different devices may produce images with different color temperatures, and the illumination conditions can vary. Our method of color tuning is simple: we shift each of the RGB channels of a fundus image to a precalculated mean and truncate the values above 255, as follows:

$$\begin{cases} R_i = \min\left\{ \dfrac{R_i}{\text{mean}(R)} \cdot r^*, 255 \right\} \\[2mm] G_i = \min\left\{ \dfrac{G_i}{\text{mean}(G)} \cdot g^*, 255 \right\}, \\[2mm] B_i = \min\left\{ \dfrac{B_i}{\text{mean}(B)} \cdot b^*, 255 \right\} \end{cases} \tag{4.1}$$

where R, G, B represent the RGB channels of the fundus image being processed, R_i, G_i, B_i represent each pixel value in the corresponding channel, and r^*, g^*, b^* are mean values of the RGB channels calculated from over 1000 fundus images that have been captured well with illumination.

This color normalization method is direct and effective, for example, the rightmost fundus image in Fig. 4.4 was enhanced significantly after color normalization. Another advantage of this method

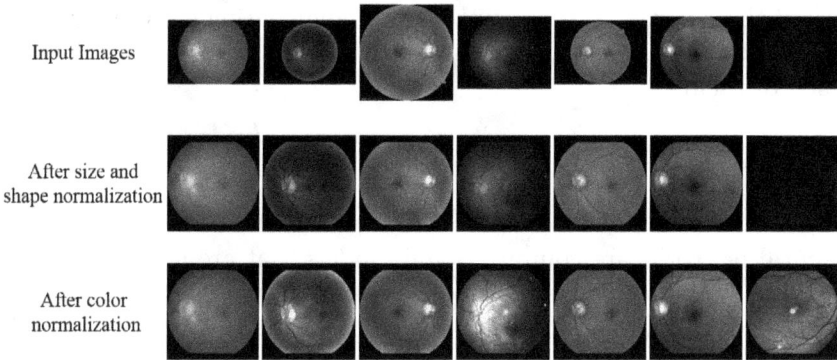

Fig. 4.4. The preprocessing pipeline.

is that it ensures that the total input values of each channel are approximately the same for different fundus images, thus providing the learning model with a more stable input range, benefiting such models as neural networks.

The overall pipeline for preprocessing is shown in Fig. 4.4, illustrated with several sample images throughout the pipeline.

4.5.2 *Augmentation*

Having sufficient training data is the key to training a neural network successfully; unfortunately, this requirement is seldom satisfied in most neural network applications. For medical imaging applications, the lack of data is more significant because of the cost of the annotations and because of the imbalance in the occurrence between diseases. To mitigate shortages in data and fully utilize the data that are available, certain data augmentation techniques must be carried out; in our experiment, we used the Augmentator software package (Bloice *et al.*, 2017). Specifically, we augmented our data through the following means:

- flip the image horizontally,
- flip the image vertically,
- randomly rotate the image in the range of [−25, 25] degrees,
- randomly zoom in or out in the range of [0.85, 1.15],
- randomly distort the image.

All of these methods were combined for augmenting each image, and
a probability of 0.5 was used to determine whether or not to perform
each of them.

4.6   Model

Neural networks are computational models that are formed by connecting simple computational units, called neurons, in certain patterns. They can, in principle, mimic behaviors of any given function if
there are enough neurons. CNNs are a special type of neural network
that was proposed by LeCun in 1990 (LeCun *et al.*, 1990). Because
of their superior performance on image-oriented tasks, they are now
the mainstream model for image-related tasks. Generally, a CNN contains three basic components: the convolutional layers, the in-place
activation operation, and the pooling layers. For classification tasks,
there may be several fully connected layers and a classification layer
at the end.

Formally, given an input $X \in \Re^{c \times m \times n}$, which is commonly an
image or a feature map of c channels and $m \times n$ size, a convolutional
layer computes a function f of X, which gives a 2-D matrix X' such
that

$$X' = f(X) = b + \sum_{j=0}^{c} W_j * X_j, \qquad (4.2)$$

where $W \in \Re^{c \times K \times K}$ is the convolution kernel of shape $c \times K \times K$,
b is the bias term, and $*$ denotes a 2-D cross-correlation operator.
A max pooling layer performs down-sampling on a given input image
or feature map by dividing the input into small patches in a sliding
window manner and computing the maximum of each patch. The
max operation can be replaced by the average or min operation,
giving different types of pooling layers. For the in-place activation
operation, a nonlinear function is used; a common choice for CNNs
is the Rectified Linear Unit (ReLU) function:

$$ReLU(x) = \begin{cases} 0 & \text{if } x < 0, \\ x & \text{otherwise.} \end{cases} \qquad (4.3)$$

For the convolutional layer and pooling layer, the sliding window on
the input can slide in an overlapping or non-overlapping manner, but

in common practice, convolutional layers are overlapping and pooling layers are non-overlapping. By interlacing convolutional layers and pooling layers, a CNN of arbitrary depth can be built. But, it is generally difficult to find a structure that works optimally for a given task.

Various CNN structures have been proposed, starting from Lenet in 1998 (LeCun *et al.*, 1998). Important breakthroughs in network structures include the Alex network (Krizhevsky *et al.*, 2012), the VGG network (Simonyan and Zisserman, 2014), the ResNet (He *et al.*, 2016b), and the Inception network (Szegedy *et al.*, 2015). Many variants have been derived from each of these typical structures. The Inception network and its derivatives are among the best image classification models and are widely used in different applications. We use the Inception-V3 network as our base model. The detailed structure of this network is given in Table 4.2. The parameters for each layer are denoted (kernel size, stride, and number of channels) for convolutional layers and (type, kernel size, and stride) for pooling layers in the Layer Configuration column. The shape of the data that pass through the network is denoted (channels, width, and height) in the Data Shape column. All convolution layers in the network are followed by a batch norm and an activation calculation and are thus omitted from the table. The Inception A/B/C/D/E modules are blocks that combine convolution layers with different kernel sizes. When using this base model directly, the output units in the last softmax output layer are reduced to four as we only have four degrees of DR severity.

We note that some microaneurysms and exudates can be really small in their size. So, when a fundus image is resized to a size of 299 by 299 pixels (the size commonly used by mainstream CNN models for image classification), small lesions in the image may be decreased to one or two pixels, making them harder to be detected. To mitigate this problem, we further propose a model for processing larger-size fundus images. Specifically, in the first step of preprocessing, we resize the fundus images to 600 by 600 pixels, then we cut each image into four 300 by 300 pieces, and feed these pieces into four different Inception-V3 models. In the end, we concatenate the features of the global average pooling layers from the four Inception-V3 models into one vector and feed this vector to a softmax output layer. We will denote this model as Inception@4 in the rest of this paper,

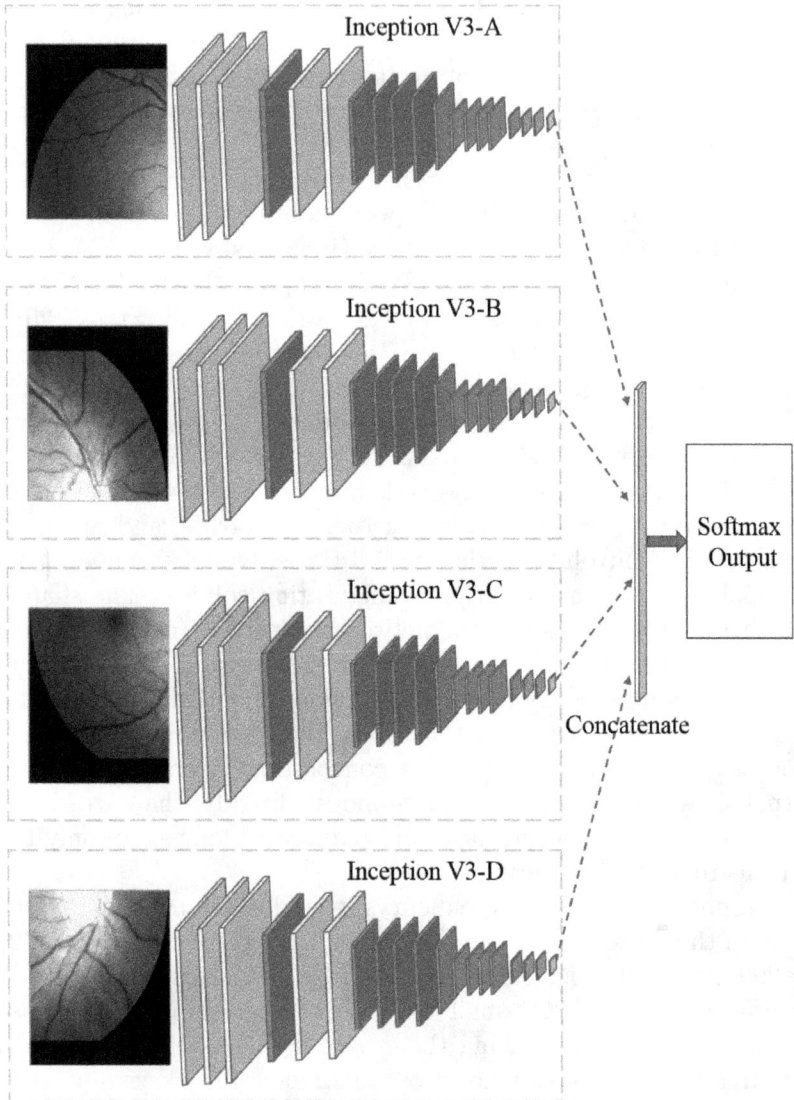

Fig. 4.5. The structure of Inception@4.

and the structure of this model is illustrated in Fig. 4.5. Since the area of the image is enlarged four times, it is easier to detect small lesions in this larger image. Compared to applying an Inception-V3 model directly on a 600 by 600 image, there are three advantages of this strategy. First, more free parameters can give the model better capacity. Second, the four models can focus on different locations of a fundus image and learn location-related lesions, such as diabetic macular edema. Third, since the original Inception-V3 model is designed for images of 299 by 299 pixels, when the input image is enlarged too much, the feature maps inside the model will be enlarged too, thus the depth of the model may no longer be optimal. In the experimental results part, we can see that this strategy improves the grading accuracy and the recall rate compared to the original Inception-V3 model.

As mentioned before, the data we have at hand are very limited compared to the tremendous amount of model parameters. To mitigate this problem, we have already used several data augmentation techniques. Another popular technique aiming at data shortage is transfer learning, i.e., transfer knowledge from domains with sufficient data to domains with insufficient data. There are many ways for doing transfer learning. For example, one can map the data from different domains to one common space and use the mapped samples as training data, or use the samples from different domains by assigning different weights. However, the most popular and ready-to-use technique is to use parameters of a model trained on problems that have sufficient data for model initialization. The purpose of this initialization is to provide the model a good starting point and avoid bad local minima. In our work, we take this approach, the parameters of models that have been pretrained on the ImageNet (Deng *et al.*, 2009) dataset are used for initialization of the networks.

4.7   Experiments

4.7.1   *Experimental setup*

We separate our data randomly into a training set and a test set at a ratio of 4:1; fundus images that are captured on each eye (one or two images per eye) are treated as a single sample. Random separation is carried out five times independently to prevent poor randomization. This results in five pairs of training and test sets. Because we separate the data based on a case rather than an image, the number

Table 4.2.   Network structure of Inception-V3 network.

Layer index	Layer type	Layer Layer configuration	Data shape
0	Data	—	(3,299,299)
1	Convolution	$(3 \times 3, 2 \times 2, 32)$	(32,149,149)
2	Convolution	$(3 \times 3, 1 \times 1, 32)$	(32,147,147)
3	Convolution	$(3 \times 3, 1 \times 1, 64)$	(64,147,147)
4	Pooling	$(\text{max}, 3 \times 3, 2 \times 2)$	(64,73,73)
5	Convolution	$(1 \times 1, 1 \times 1, 80)$	(80,73,73)
6	Convolution	$(3 \times 3/1 \times 1, 192)$	(192,71,71)
7	Pooling	$(\text{max}, 3 \times 3, 2 \times 2)$	(192,35,35)
8	Inception A	—	(256,35,35)
9	Inception A	—	(288,35,35)
10	Inception A	—	(288,35,35)
11	Inception B	—	(768,17,17)
12	Inception C	—	(768,17,17)
13	Inception C	—	(768,17,17)
14	Inception C	—	(768,17,17)
15	Inception C	—	(768,17,17)
16	Inception D	—	(1280,8,8)
17	Inception E	—	(2048,8,8)
18	Inception E	—	(2048,8,8)
19	Pooling	$(\text{avg}, 8 \times 8, 1 \times 1)$	(2048,1,1)
20	Softmax Output	—	4

of samples in each category varies slightly in different training/test set pairs. The statistics of each training/test set pair are listed in Table 4.3.

We evaluate the Inception-V3 and Inception@4 models on each of these dataset pairs; several mainstream models, such as the ResNet model and the VGG model, are evaluated as a comparison. The evaluation metrics we use are as follows. First, we calculate the 4-classification accuracy of the models that are evaluated. Because the rate of missed diagnoses is important for clinical applications, we further calculate the precision and recall rate of the models, for the calculation of these two metrics, the three degrees besides normal are considered as a with DR degree. The precision of a model indicates the reliability of the model diagnosing a patient as ill, and the recall rate reflects the sensitivity of a model to the disease being diagnosed.

Table 4.3.   Training/Test set statistics.

Dataset	Set	Normal	Moderate	Heavy	Severe	Total
Dataset 1	Training	1513	760	975	321	3569
	test	385	190	247	85	907
Dataset 2	Training	1518	758	970	322	3568
	test	380	192	252	84	908
Dataset 3	Training	1515	759	964	320	3558
	test	383	191	258	86	918
Dataset 4	Training	1515	759	965	327	3566
	test	383	191	257	79	910
Dataset 5	Training	1518	760	976	318	3572
	test	380	190	246	88	904

These metrics are calculated as

$$P = \frac{TP}{TP + FP}, \tag{4.4}$$

and

$$R = \frac{TP}{FN + TP}, \tag{4.5}$$

where TP, FP, and FN denote True Positive, False Positive, and False Negative, respectively.

All of these evaluations are carried out independently. The platform we use to conduct the experiments is a workstation with 2 Xeon E5-2620 CPUs, 2 Tesla K40 GPUs, and 64G of RAM. The network implementation is done using the MXNET package (Chen *et al.*, 2015).

4.7.2   *Details of learning*

During training, we use a batch size of 32; for the Inception@4 model, the batch size is reduced to 4 since it requires more GPU RAM; the optimizer we use is an Adam optimizer with a learning rate of 1e-05, the weight decay rate is set as 0.2 to prevent overfitting, and other parameters of the optimizer are set using the default values in MXNET, i.e., beta1=0.9, beta2=0.999, and epsilon=1e-08.

Table 4.4.   The results of the models evaluated.

	Accuracy (%)	Precision (%)	Recall (%)
Resnet-18	87.61	95.76	92.52
Resnet-101	87.26	95.63	92.48
VGG-19	85.50	94.00	93.01
Inception-V3	88.35	**96.51**	92.41
Inception@4	**88.72**	95.77	**94.84**

Note: The bold numbers indicate the best performance.

All parameters in these models are initialized using models pre-trained on the ImageNet dataset. For parameters not in the pre-trained models, i.e., the parameters of the output layers, we use a Xavier initializer with a magnitude of 1 for initialization.

During training, we found that the I/O operation for reading the images from the disk takes a lot of time. In order to reduce this time, we set up a separate process to cache all the preprocessed images in the RAM; the training process can then retrieve each mini-batch of data from the caching process. This strategy boosts the training significantly and is particularly useful when a number of models need to be evaluated simultaneously for many times.

4.7.3   *Results*

The evaluation results (averaged over five datasets) for each model are listed in Table 4.4. The Inception-V3 model and the adapted Inception@4 model surpass all other models. It is notable that by classifying more Normal samples (together with samples with Mild DR) as Mild DR, the recall rate of VGG-19 is 0.6% higher than that of Inception-V3, however this is at the cost of 2.51% of precision and 2.85% overall accuracy. For a similar reason, the Inception@4 model has a lower precision rate than the Inception-V3 model, however, the increase in accuracy and recall is more significant and preferable.

4.7.4   *Visualization*

The success of neural network models is largely based on their revolutionary performance and simplicity in the model setup. The only requirement for training a neural network is a dataset of input–output pairs; no feature engineering is required, and the network will automatically learn the mapping between inputs and outputs. This black box character renders neural networks easy to use; as a trade-off, the explainability of neural networks is poor. Much effort has been made to demystify how neural networks function. For the CNN models that were used in the image classification problem, many techniques have been proposed to visualize what the model really learns; such approaches include the occlusion test, feature visualization, deconvolutional networks (Zeiler and Fergus, 2014), and classification activation map (CAM) (Zhou *et al.*, 2016). Here, we used the CAM method for the visualization analysis. A CAM is obtained by weighting the feature maps before the global average pooling layer at the end of the network. By projecting the weights of the output layer onto the feature maps, the contribution of each region that is activated in these feature maps can be combined to indicate the regions in the input that count toward the prediction.

In Fig. 4.6, we highlight representative results that were obtained using CAM on the trained Inception@4 model. For the CAM and Combined image columns, four patches from the four submodels are combined. We can see clearly that for these images, the model learns to focus on the main lesions during the classification process.

To further analyze the performance of the trained models, we plotted the confusion matrices of the Inception@4 model on five test sets in Fig. 4.7. From the confusion matrices, we can see that most of the misclassifications lay between adjacent categories, indicating that such samples are hard to separate for the model. We conjecture that this is because the progression of DR is continuous; thus, the category to which a patient belongs in certain stages is ambiguous. One important issue we must consider is the impact of false negative diagnoses. From the confusion matrices, we can see that all false negative diagnoses are the ones that should be graded as Moderate. From Table 4.1, we can see that the suggested treatment for a Moderate DR patient is recheck in 6 months, and the suggested treatment for a diabetic patient without DR is recheck in 12 months. Thus, for the false negative diagnoses, delayed treatment of 6 months can be caused. From the confusion matrices, we can estimate that the rate of Moderate DR to be graded as Normal is 14.25%, and we can also see that the probability of Moderate DR change into high-risk PDR within one year is at most 8.1% (Ophthalmoscopy and Levels, 2002). Thus, the impact of such false negative diagnoses is limited.

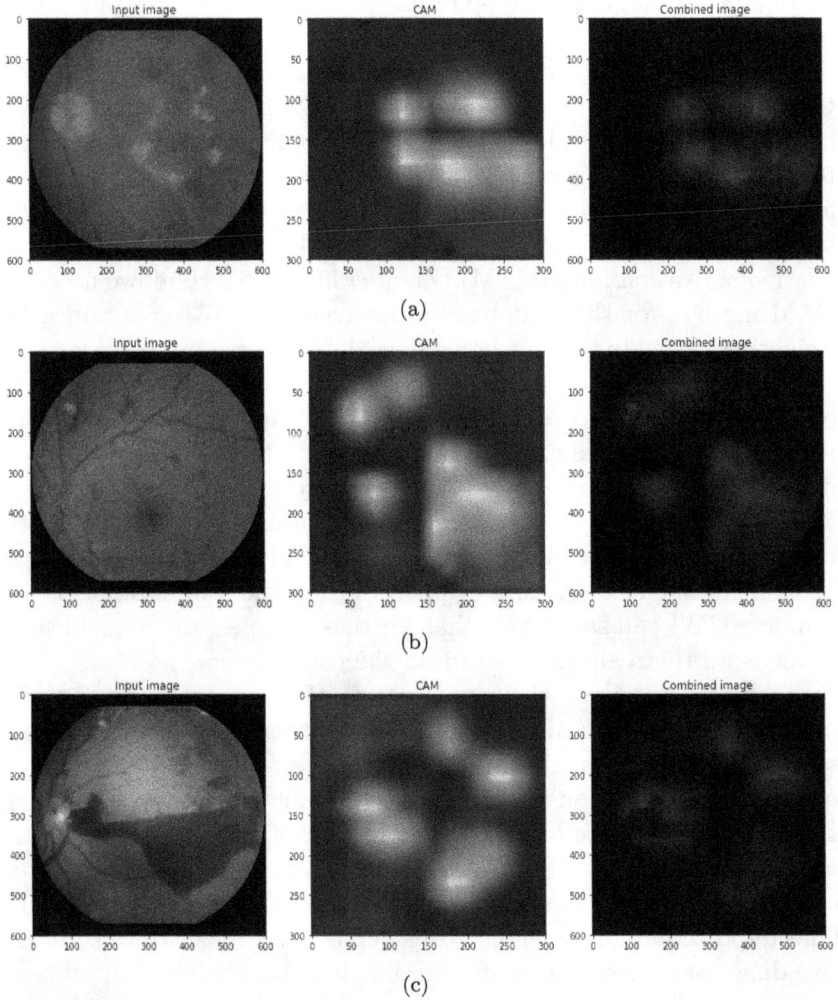

Fig. 4.6. Typical results for CAM on the trained Inception@4 model.

4.8 Model Deployment and Clinical Evaluation

To meet the requirements of clinical applications, we have built a system that diagnoses DR via the Internet. The models[1] are first

---

[1]Currently, we ensemble five Inception-V3 models on the cloud rather than five Inception@4 models for the sake of saving GPU RAM.

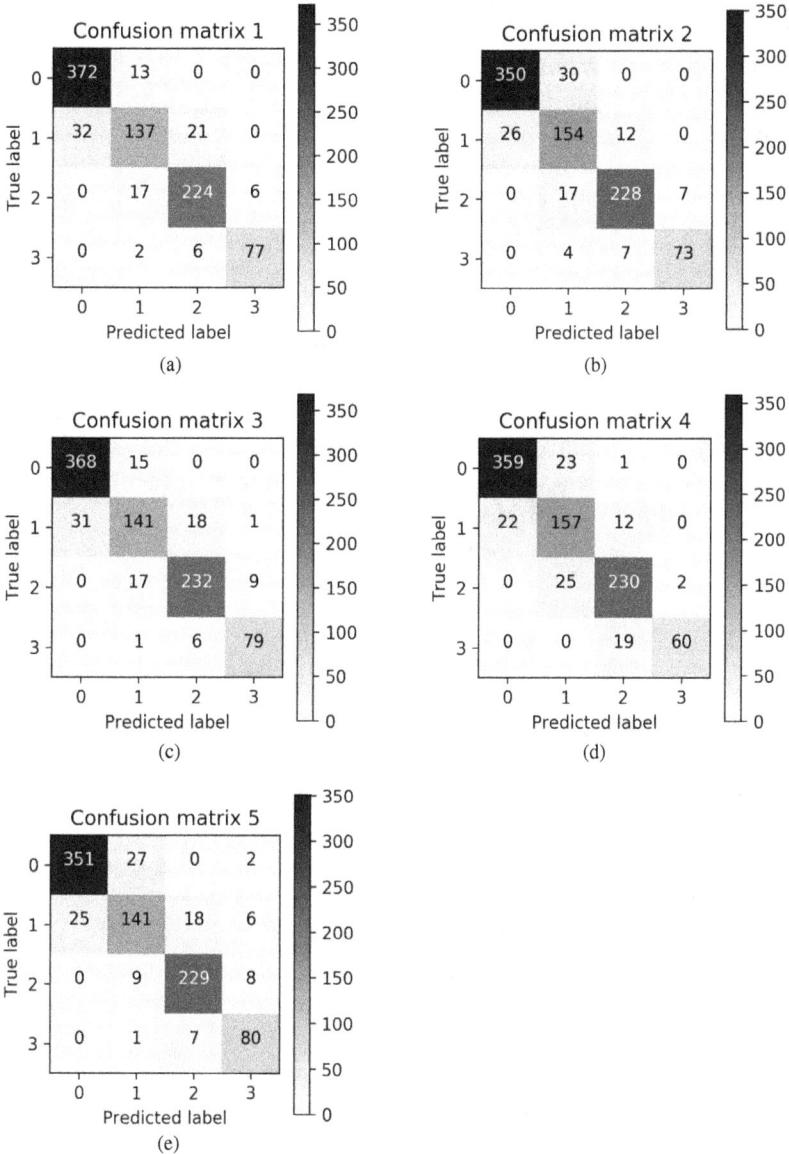

Fig. 4.7. The confusion matrix of Inception@4 network on each test set. (a) Confusion matrix on dataset 1, (b) confusion matrix on dataset 2, (c) confusion matrix on dataset 3, (d) confusion matrix on dataset 4, and (e) confusion matrix on dataset 5.

deployed on a cloud computing platform to compute the diagnosis; then, a web server is deployed to wrap the models and provide a user interface to users from different hospitals via the Internet. The pilot runs are carried out in four hospitals in different locations. During the pilot runs, users from these hospitals upload images to the system and get diagnosis results from the system. In the backstage, ophthalmologists from the annotation team login to the system and retrieve all uploaded cases. Then, all uploaded cases are annotated again by the ophthalmologists. The annotation results are then treated as the ground truth to judge the performance of the system. Thus far, the diagnosis consistency between the system and ophthalmologists reaches 91.8% (259 out of 282 valid diagnoses, all testing cases new to the models), demonstrating the reliable performance of the system in a clinical environment. Similar to results in the experimental section, all false negative cases are cases that should be graded as Moderate which require no urgent treatments.

4.9   Conclusion

The huge population of diabetic patients and the prevalence of DR among them have fostered a great demand for automatic DR diagnosis systems. So far, a lot of achievements have been made and satisfactory results have been achieved in many subproblems like vessel segmentation and lesion detection. However, these results are obtained on datasets relatively small and are steps away from real-world applications.

For clinical applications, systems that can give DR severity directly are more favorable and practical. However, current results for multi-class severity grading are still not good enough for clinical application. In this work, we investigated the automatic grading of DR using deep neural networks. We proposed a novel dataset that is moderate in size and annotated with a new labeling scheme that is more useful for clinical practice. We proposed a preprocessing pipeline to change fundus images into a uniform format. We used the Inception-V3 network and a proposed modification of it as our diagnostic models and evaluated the performance of them with several mainstream CNN models. The experimental results demonstrate the efficiency of the models in diagnosing DR. Visualization and analysis of the trained models provide insights into how the models make diagnoses using given fundus images and justify the diagnostic ability of the models from a different viewpoint. For clinical applications, the trained models are deployed on a cloud computing platform and provide pilot diagnostic services to several hospitals via the Internet. The performance of the system in the clinical evaluation demonstrates the efficiency of this work. In the future, data from more equipment will be included, and a broader pilot study will be launched. The accumulated data will be further used to improve the accuracy of the models.

Chapter 5

Automated Identification and Grading System of Diabetic Retinopathy Using Deep Neural Networks

Diabetic retinopathy (DR) is a major cause of human vision loss worldwide. Slowing down the progress of the disease requires early screening. However, the clinical diagnosis of DR presents a considerable challenge in low-resource settings where few ophthalmologists are available to care for all patients with diabetes. In this study, an automated DR identification and grading system called DeepDR is proposed. DeepDR directly detects the presence and severity of DR from fundus images via transfer learning and ensemble learning. It comprises a set of state-of-the-art neural networks based on combinations of popular convolutional neural networks and customized standard deep neural networks. The DeepDR system is developed by constructing a high-quality dataset of DR medical images and then labeled by clinical ophthalmologists. We further explore the relationship between the number of ideal component classifiers and the number of class labels, as well as the effects of different combinations of component classifiers on the best integration performance to construct an optimal model. We evaluate the models on the basis of validity and reliability using nine metrics. Results show that the identification model performs best with a sensitivity of 97.5%, a specificity of 97.7%, and an area under the curve of 97.7%. Meanwhile, the grading model achieves a sensitivity of 98.1% and a specificity of 98.9%. On the basis of the above methods, DeepDR can detect DR satisfactorily. Experiment results indicate the importance and effectiveness of the ideal number and combinations of component classifiers in relation to model performance. DeepDR provides reproducible and consistent detection results with high sensitivity and specificity instantaneously. Hence, this work provides ophthalmologists with insights into the diagnostic process.

5.1 Related Works

In the past few decades, the development of automated DR pathology screening has made encouraging progress. From an application perspective, computer-aided detection (CADe) algorithms and computer-aided diagnosis (CADx) algorithms can be viewed as typical representatives in the field. CADe detects lesions at the pixel level with manual segmentations (Winder *et al.*, 2009). On the basis of the detected lesions, CADx detects pathologies at the image level (Abràmoff *et al.*, 2010).

5.1.1 *Traditional methods for DR diagnosis*

From a methodological perspective, automated screening for DR has long focused on pattern recognition or traditional machine learning algorithms. Walter *et al.* (2002) created efficient algorithms for detecting optic disc and exudates; these algorithms yielded a mean sensitivity of 92.8% and a mean predictive value of 92.4% on 30 images. Niemeijer *et al.* (2007) developed a machine learning system capable of detecting exudates, cotton wool spots, and drusen; their system can differentiate among 300 color images, and its reporting performance approaches that of retinal experts. Faust *et al.* (2012) contributed an important and valuable review of algorithms used for extractions of these features from retinopathy images; they also discussed some reported classification systems. Akram *et al.* (2014) presented a hybrid classifier comprising classifiers that could be used to detect all types of non-proliferative DR (NPDR) lesions and grade different stages of NPDR on the basis of a Gaussian mixture model and m-Medoids; whereas the area under the curve (AUC) values of m-Mediods and Gaussian mixture model are 97.7% and 96.3%, respectively, that of the hybrid classifier achieves reaches 98.1%. Viswanatha *et al.* (2018) employed the fuzzy c-means clustering method on a dataset consisting of 100 images to identify the exact region of DR and reported an accuracy of 99.01%, a sensitivity of 98.38%, and a specificity of 96.36%.

Some obvious shortcomings of these techniques include the following: First, they focus on feature engineering, such that the extraction of features must be specified by experts; fulfilling such requirement is a time-consuming process and increases the burden on clinicians. Second, they show limited scope because the studies present results that were derived from small databases; thus, the generalization and robustness of systems are limited to a certain extent. Third, the early clinical symptoms of DR are not always obvious, and the sizes of some lesions are insufficient to attract the attention of some graders. Hence, questions arise with regard to the accurate extraction of lesion features and comprehensive diagnosis. This approach is thus transformed into a complex vision issue, although this type of error is relatively understandable. Therefore, one of the ultimate goals of artificial intelligence is to automate this process of feature engineering as much as possible.

5.1.2 *Deep learning for DR diagnosis*

Deep learning, especially CNNs, provides powerful support to alleviate the aforementioned problems. Models trained by deep learning can discern subtle local features directly from retinopathy images without human effort or specific domain knowledge.

Litjens *et al.* (2017) contributed an important survey regarding the use of deep learning in image classification, object detection, segmentation, registration, and other tasks. They summarized over 300 contributions to the field, most of which appeared in 2016. All top algorithms in the Kaggle machine learning competition (Kaggle, 2016) in 2015 used CNNs to support an automated DR detection system. Benson *et al.* (2018) repurposed an existing deep network for DR screening via transfer learning and other pre-preprocessing techniques on 979 clinical cases; the repurposed deep network achieves a 95% AUC for identifying severe DR with equal sensitivity and specificity of 90%. Gargeya and Leng (2017) developed a data-driven deep learning algorithm capable of classifying fundus images as healthy or not; this algorithm identifies relevant cases with high reliability. Gulshan *et al.* (2016) created a deep learning-trained algorithm for detecting referable diabetic retinopathy (RDR) in two separate datasets of 9,963 and 1,748 images; the algorithm achieved high sensitivity (97.5% and 96.1%) and specificity (93.4% and 93.9%) when applied to the two datasets. A study by researchers at Stanford University (Tamkin *et al.*, 2013) used the Inception-V3 model via transfer learning techniques; the approach achieves 72.96% accuracy in detection of RDR and 92.59% accuracy in detection of stage PDR. Pratt *et al.* (2016) designed a CNN network that enables a classifier to predict the exact DR stage of the sample for a five-class DR detection task. The proposed technique achieves 75% accuracy, 30% sensitivity, and 95% specificity.

5.2   Dataset

5.2.1   *Materials*

In our study, macula-centered retinal fundus images were taken from the Sichuan Academy of Medical Sciences and Sichuan Provincial People's Hospital between September 2017 and May 2018. The original data comprising 13,767 images of 1872 patients were collected from three sources: ophthalmology, endocrinology, and physical examination centers (Fig. 5.1). In general, almost all patients from the ophthalmology department were diagnosed with DR, and nearly two-thirds of the patients from the endocrinology department had DR; the data from the physical examination center showed no DR symptoms among patients. As almost all patients from ophthalmology department had DR, two types of images, namely, retinal color fundus photographs and fluorescein angiography fundus photographs (pharmacological pupil dilation), were required, and two or more photographs with a 45° view were captured per eye. This project aims to screen preoperative fundus retinal images and to diagnose the degree of lesions. Therefore, all fluorescence contrast images and postoperative fundus images, that is, 9934 images in 1229 patients, were excluded. For the patients from the endocrinology

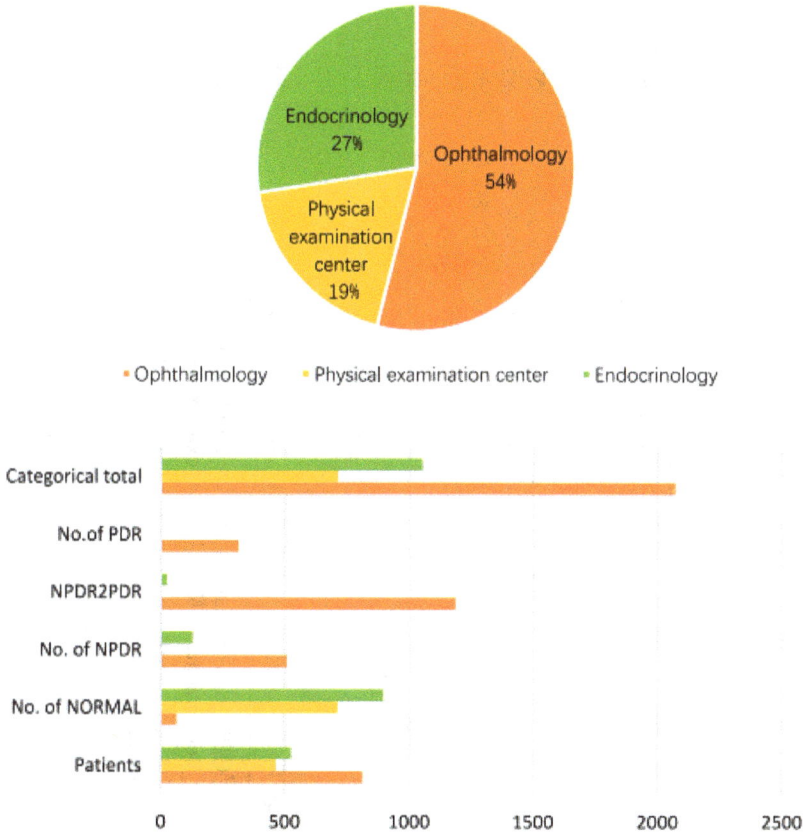

Fig. 5.1. Characteristics of the dataset for DR.

and physical examination centers, only fundus photos of each eye were taken. Further detailed statistics of the dataset are shown in Table 5.1.

5.2.2 Grading standard

Although ETDRS has indispensable reference value for our labeling work, some challenges remained in the grading of DR. First, the interpretation for the reference criteria primarily depends on the ophthalmologist's experience of reading images with reference

Table 5.1. Summary of Training and Validation datasets for DR.

Source	Camera	Assessors	Patients	Images	Images/Eye	Normal	Npdr	Npdr2pdr	Pdr	Total[1]
Training										
OPH[2]	Canon	(1,2)[3]	613	1669	2~6[4]	50	421	953	245	1669
PEC[5]	Canon	(1,2)	379	575	1~2[6]	575	0	0	0	575
END[7]	Kowa	(1,2)	409	818	2	696	100	19	3	818
total_t[8]			1401	3062		1321(0.43)	521(0.17)	972(0.32)	248(0.08)	3062
Validation										
OPH	Canon	(1,2)	199	401	2~6	12	87	234	68	401
PEC	Canon	(1,2)	86	136	1~2[6]	136	0	0	0	136
END	Kowa	(1,2)	117	234	2	200	27	6	1	234
total_v[9]			402	771		348(0.45)	114(0.15)	240(0.31)	69(0.09)	771
Total[10]			1803	3833		1619	635	1212	317	3833

Notes: [1]Total: total of images in the department, [2]OPH: ophthalmology, [3](1,2): 2 ophthalmologists, 1 retinal specialist, [4]2~6: number of fundus photographs taken per eye per patient, [5]PEC: physical examination center, [6]1~2: some patients had only 1 images per eye, [7]END: endocrinology, [8]total_t: categorical total of training dataset, [9]total_v: categorical total of validation dataset, [10]Total: categorical total of training and validation.

to the guidelines and is thus qualitative rather than quantitative; thus, the assessment of severity has a degree of subjectivity. Second, most patients with DR in China often neglect this disease and thus fail to secure timely interventions; as a result, their cases become aggravated, with symptoms being frequently considered as intermediate to severe NPDR and early PDR. Third, because the transition period above has similar clinical manifestations, the recommended treatment for them, according to the ETDRS, is the same. This situation is also reflected in cases ranging from mild NPDR to moderate NPDR.

Therefore, we classified severity into four levels: normal, NPDR, NPDR2PDR, and PDR. This annotation strategy was used in our four-class classification task.

5.2.3 *Manual grading*

All images of the dataset were assessed in stages as the data volume accumulated. The graders included one retinal specialist with more than 27 years of experience in DR research and two seasoned ophthalmologists with more than five years of experience in clinical diagnosis and treatment. The entire grading process was divided into three steps. First, the annotators indicated whether a given image was of sufficient quality for grading. Second, the quality of the image was deemed insufficient when it became difficult or impossible to make a confident assessment regarding the characteristics of DR. Then, the image was categorized as normal (absence of DR) and abnormal (presence of DR). Third, the severity of DR in the abnormal images was annotated.

The grading reliability of each image was measured by cross-validation (checking others' grading results per image for every grader). First, almost all patients from the ophthalmology department were found with DR; hence, we used two types of images per eye: retinal color fundus photographs and fluorescein angiography fundus photographs (pharmacological pupil dilation). The fundus images labeled with inconsistency were corrected using the original diagnosis reports with corresponding photographs of fluorescein angiography because accuracy ultimately came from fluorescent photography. Meanwhile, only retinal color fundus photos were taken from the patients from the endocrine and physical examination centers. Disagreements were re-examined and resolved via discussion. If no consensus was reached, arbitration was performed by the retinal expert to generate final grading.

5.2.4   *Preprocessing of retinal images*

Given the complexity of the retina structure, the characteristics of DR were easily confused with those of other eye diseases. Moreover, we observed a range of imaging noise, such as black space on either side of the eye, low contrast, blurred lens, or insufficient light. As a result, some minute lesions could not be accurately identified within the poor photographs. Therefore, some preprocessing was necessary. Figure 7.1 shows some examples of poor-quality data.

First, an algorithm was devised to remove the invalid areas of black space by cropping a fixed number of pixels from each of the four sides of each image while avoiding a large amount of computational overhead caused by the black space. Second, the images exhibited resolutions in the range of 1631×1879 to 1823×1650; we standardized the resolution by downsizing all images to a uniform size in accordance with the input requirements of specific models. Furthermore, for measuring the light intensity at each pixel in a single image, we converted all images to grayscale. For the images with excessively bright or dark background and foreground, we used histogram equalization (HE) to improve the visual effects of the images and to discover hidden messages. To improve local contrast and enhance edge definition in each image region, we used adaptive HE, which was initially proposed by Stark (2000), Stark and Fitzgerald (1994), as a part of the preprocessing steps. Mathematically, the adaptive HE can be written as follows:

$$f_c(u, v) = q(u - v, \alpha) - \beta q(u - v, 1) + \beta u q(d, \alpha),$$

$$q(d, \alpha) = \frac{1}{2} \sin(d) \, |2d|^\alpha,$$

(5.1)

where $0 \leq \alpha$ and $\beta \leq 1$, and we set $\alpha = \beta$. f_c is an accumulation function, and HE is given if $\alpha = 0$. These equations are explained in detail in Stark and Fitzgerald (1994).

For dark images, we provided a contrast stretching algorithm to enhance the contrast effect of each area of the image. This algorithm was performed by using the following equation:

$$I(x,y) = \frac{I(x,y) - I_{\min}}{I_{\max} - I_{\min}} \times 255, \tag{5.2}$$

where $I(x,y)$ is the gray value of a pixel in the original image and $I_{\min}$ and $I_{\max}$ are the real minimum and maximum grayscale values of the original image, respectively.

5.2.5 *Performance comparison*

Figure 5.2 shows some examples of the preprocessing in our dataset. The comparative experiment was executed via Xception. The model performed well in the binary task. The model was trained via resizing only and no other preprocessing. Then, it was compared with the models trained with all the preprocessing methods. The accuracy of the model without preprocessing reached 94.79% until 300 epochs. This model's accuracy did not exceed such level even after fine-tuning. By contrast, the model with preprocessing converged well after 220 epochs and achieved an accuracy of 95.68%. This accuracy rate improved to 97.15% after fine-tuning (Fig. 5.8). Figure 5.3 and Table 5.5 provide further details.

5.2.6 *Data augmentation*

The amount of PDR only accounted for 9% of the total data (Table 5.1), and the inter-grader variability was serious in the pathological features. The model had difficulties in learning the characteristics of PDR, and PDR was overidentified as NPDR2PDR. Therefore, we used data augmentation technology, such as random rotation by $0°-180°$, random horizontal or vertical flips, to enhance the size of the training set in real time. Generally, augmented images retained the major features of their original images. Therefore, the technologies ensured that the training set was expanded while the images were not copied completely.

(a) Normal and DR level

(b) Normal and DR level

(c) Example images of data preprocessing

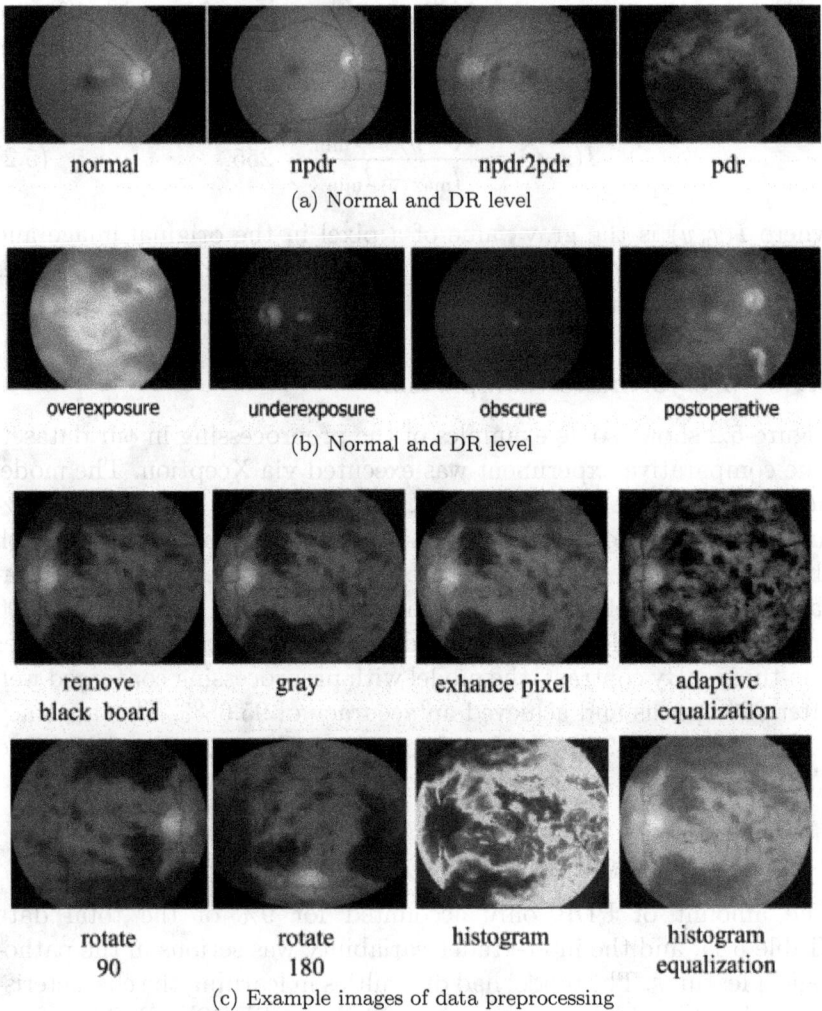

Fig. 5.2.   Example images of poor quality and preprocessing in the dataset.

5.3   Model and Methodology

5.3.1   *Aim and objective*

The following two aims motivated this study and were realized with corresponding ensemble models that were designed in this work.

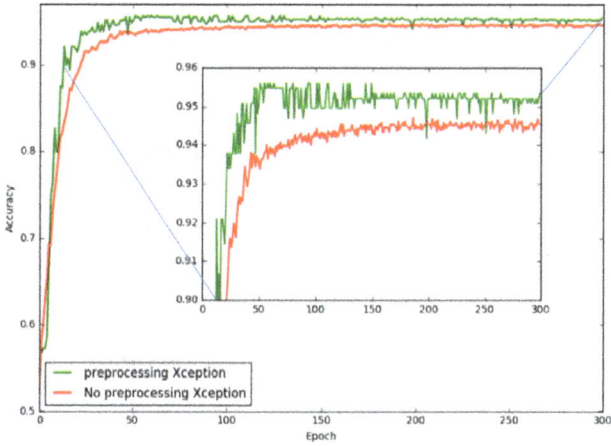

(a) Comparison of accuracy

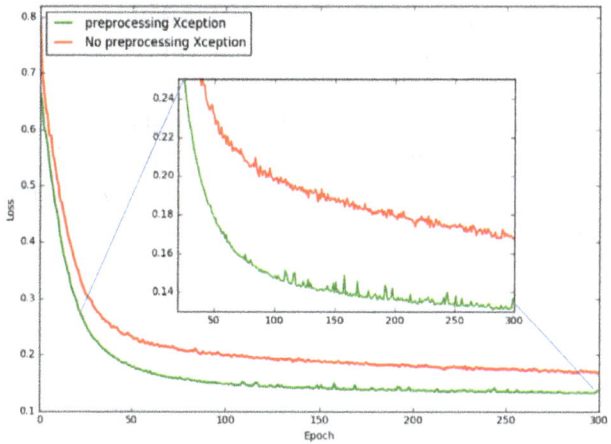

(b) Comparison of loss

Fig. 5.3. The comparison before and after preprocessing of the identification system.

(1) **To build an early DR automatic screening system:** This aim is a binary classification task to identify the presence of DR. Currently, the manual DR screening method is labor intensive and suffers from inconsistencies across sites (Goh *et al.*, 2016); moreover, the number of people who can master DR treatment skills is still small among most grassroots health workers. Therefore, the first task was primarily applied to communities at the grassroots level

because patients with DR may be identified timely and referred to ophthalmology for further diagnosis and treatment while potentially alleviating the burden for ophthalmologists.

(2) **To build an automatic grading system:** This aim is a multi-classification task to predict the level of DR severity. The grading system was primarily used in hospitals to provide ophthalmologists with auxiliary diagnostic references while avoiding human subjectivity.

5.3.2 *Architecture and strategy of ensemble model*

In this study, "learner", "basic learner", "component classifier", and "component" refer to an independent neural network used in an ensemble.

Several components comprised a corresponding ensemble model. Each component was a two-part neural network. The first part was a feature extractor comprising a pretraining model that was initialized via transfer learning which involved the removal of the top layer. The second part was a classifier that made predictions on the basis of the aforementioned features; it was realized by a customized stand deep neural network with training from scratch.

5.3.3 *Ensemble strategy*

Many studies have largely realized ensemble methods with many components at the expense of time and memory. Therefore, the number of component classifiers to be included in the ensemble is an important issue in integration model experiments (Tsoumakas *et al.*, 2008). The issue further triggers deep thinking, namely, the choice of combination method and the training mechanism of components, which largely characterize the ensemble method (Hernández-Lobato *et al.*, 2013; Bonab and Can, 2016, 2019). The former indicates which learners can be combined, whereas the latter describes how to combine them.

For "which learners", extensive literature has shown that the performance of the overall classifier can be enhanced if a not-so-weak learner is used as a base learner (Dietterich, 2000). Meanwhile, the predictive power of a learner is closely related to its ability to extract high-quality features; thus, a high-performance premodel must be selected as the feature extractor in the bottom part of the component.

For "how to", because DNNS has high variance and low bias, the variance of models can be dramatically reduced via averaging if the models are independent (Simonyan and Zisserman, 2014; Ju *et al.*, 2018). In this work, we averaged the softmax scores of all models to solve the second issue above because these probabilities from different models might have varying output magnitudes. Comparative experiments between the averaging and max methods applied to the ensemble models were added for objectivity. The results demonstrated that the averaging method was more effective in our study (Table 5.6).

5.3.4   *Transfer learning at the first part*

Several standout CNNs that remove top layers made up the first stage of different ensembles. We used these CNNs to produce a compact feature vector representation in a DR image. In consideration of different tasks, we performed some analyses of respective CNN characteristics as follows to facilitate our selection of a strong feature extractor (learner) for each component of the ensemble.

To enhance the speed of the calculation, we used ResNet50 (He *et al.*, 2015b) and InceptionV3 (Szegedy *et al.*, 2016) as alternatives. InceptionResNetV2 (Szegedy *et al.*, 2017) was also attempted because it can make the network deep and fast by mitigating the problem of gradient disappearance using jumper connections. Similarly, Xception (Chollet, 2017) was considered as one improvement to InceptionV3 due to its ability to improve the effects of the model without increasing the complexity of the network. DenseNets (Huang *et al.*, 2017) were attractive because they can fully use the features and further reduce gradient disappearance; furthermore, they performed well in our experiments.

5.3.5   *Design of customized Standard Deep Neural Network (SDNN) at the second part*

On the basis of the specific data distributions and difficulties of the two tasks, two respective types of SDNNs were defined as component classifiers at the second stage (Fig. 7.2). Input to the SDNNs was given by the output of the feature extractors. SDNNs have the same network depth but different parameters. This faint distinction led to important changes in the prediction performance: through experiments and observations, we found that adding or removing a layer could reduce the learning capacity of the network regardless of the task. Given the similarity of designs of SDNN frameworks, we showed only the development of the SDNN model in the four-class classification task.

Notably, the feature maps from the forward layer are spatial, but they can be normalized via global average pooling (GAP). Thus, we designed a GAP layer as the first layer of the SDNN. The second layer was a fully connected layer with 2,048 hidden neurons. Proper nonlinearity is an important factor in the incremental performance of a classification model, especially for a limited dataset. Thus, we closely monitored the effects of nonlinearity between the rectified linear unit function (ReLU) and its variant, leaky rectified linear unit function (leaky ReLU), on SDNN performance. In the same condition, we conducted multiple comparison experiments and found that leaky ReLU was significantly faster than ReLU with respect to convergence and shortening of training time. According to prior literature (Bonab and Can, 2016, 2019; Dietterich, 2000), the difference may be caused by the potential disadvantage of ReLU during optimization: the gradient is 0 whenever the neuron is dead (saturated and not active). This occurrence may cause the unit to remain inactive because the gradient-based optimization algorithm does not adjust the weight of a dead neuron. Therefore, the speed of training ReLU networks is slow when gradients remain at zero. By contrast, leaky ReLU slightly adjusts the weight of dead neurons into small and non-zero gradients. On the basis of the above analysis, we applied leaky ReLU layers to the output of all inner fully connected layers, except the output layer, to achieve nonlinearity in the SDNN. The two functions of ReLU and leaky ReLU are defined in Eqs. (5.3) and (5.4), respectively.

$$h^{(i)} = \max(w^{(i)(T)}x, 0) = \begin{cases} w^{(i)T}x, & \text{if } w^{(i)T}x > 0 \\ 0, & \text{otherwise,} \end{cases} \tag{5.3}$$

$$h^{(i)} = \max(w^{(i)(T)}x, 0) = \begin{cases} w^{(i)T}x, & \text{if } w^{(i)T}x > 0 \\ 0.01w^{(i)T}x, & \text{otherwise.} \end{cases} \tag{5.4}$$

The above formulas show the similarities and differences between the two functions. The latter function may achieve a more robust gradient than the former by sacrificing sparsity.

A dropout layer was added after each dense layer. The addition can effectively omit many neurons of hidden layers during training and ensure the validity of the data; it can also mitigate or prevent data overfitting if the network shows excessive reliance on certain nodes in one layer. We updated each node with probability $p = 0.5$ while updating each layer. Then, we left it unchanged with probability $1 - p$. Following these multiple layers, the final layer was a standard softmax classifier with cross-entropy as the loss function. The softmax function took an N-dimensional vector of arbitrary real values and produced another N-dimensional vector with real values in the range $(0,1)$, thereby adding up to 1.0; each value of the output vector represented the probability that the sample belonged to each class. Cross-entropy served as a loss function that revealed the distance or degree of closeness between the true labels and the predicted labels of the network. It is defined as follows:

$$L_j = - \log \left(\frac{e^{s_j}}{\sum_{k=1}^{N} e^{s_k}} \right), \tag{5.5}$$

where N indicates the number of classes, s_j is the score for the sample label j, and s_k is the score for a particular label k. Softmax ensured that the prediction probabilities exhibited a proper probability distribution.

5.4 Experiments

5.4.1 *Configuration*

The algorithms were implemented using Keras (http://keras.io/). All experiments were performed on a high-end workstation with an Intel Xeon E5-2620 CPU and NVIDIA Tesla K40 GPU with 64GB of RAM. The dataset was split into 70% for training, 10% for validation, and 20% for testing. The configuration of the hyper-parameter and the class distributions of the two tasks are shown in Tables 5.2–5.4.

Table 5.2.　Hyper-parameter configuration.

Configuration	Value
Optimization function	RMSprop
Epoch	300(training), 100(fine turning)
Batch size	32
Learning rate	2.00E-04
Drop out	5.00E-01
Class_weight	auto
ReduceLROn Plateau	monitor='val_acc', factor=0.5, patience=10, epsilon=0.0001
EarlyStopping	monitor='val_loss', patience=15
ModelCheckpoint	monitor='val_acc', mode='auto', period=1

Table 5.3.　Class distribution and classifications report of the identification system.

	Training	Validation	Testing	
Normal	1189	132	348	
Abnormal	1567	174	423	
Total	2756	306	771	

	Precision	Recall	F1-score	Support
Normal	0.97	0.98	0.97	348
Abnormal	0.98	0.97	0.98	423
Ave/total	0.98	0.98	0.98	771

5.4.2　*Strategy*

The experiment process consisted of six steps: input data, data preprocessing, single-model feature extraction, single-model feature classification, multi-model feature fusion, and output results (Fig. 5.4–5.6). During one component development, the first phase focused on the separate pretraining of the SDNNs; the key points were the number of layers needed in each SDNN with corresponding parameters to achieve optimal performance. The second phase was to combine each preprocessing model with the corresponding SDNN model with retraining. Lastly, the component was fine-tuned by determining the suitable layer to be frozen. For convenience, each

Table 5.4.   Class distribution and classifications report of the grading system.

	Training	Validation	Testing
Normal	1189	132	348
NPDR	469	52	114
NPDR2PDR	875	97	240
PDR	224	25	69
Total	2756	306	771

	Precision	Recall	F1-score	Support
Normal	0.98	0.99	0.98	348
NPDR	0.92	0.88	0.9	114
NPDR2PDR	0.96	0.98	0.97	240
PDR	1	0.94	0.97	69
Ave/total	0.96	0.96	0.96	771

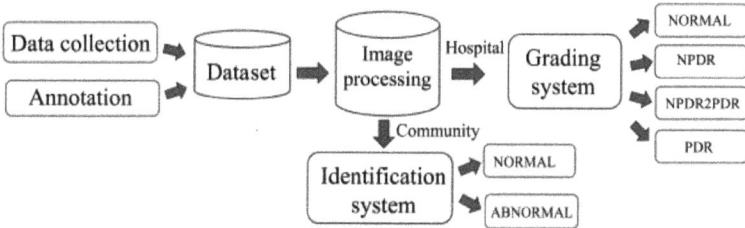

Fig. 5.4.   The flowchart of the proposed method.

component classifier was named the components' internal pretraining model.

Models were designed in parallel and independently while taking them as alternative component classifiers. The choice of the most suitable component classifier and the size of the ensemble have a great impact on the accuracy of the prediction results of the model. Therefore, we attempted rich experiments to explore the relationship among the ideal size of the ensemble model (the number of basic component classifiers), the optimal width of the ensemble model (the combination method of component classifiers), and the number of class labels for the two systems on the basis of our dataset.

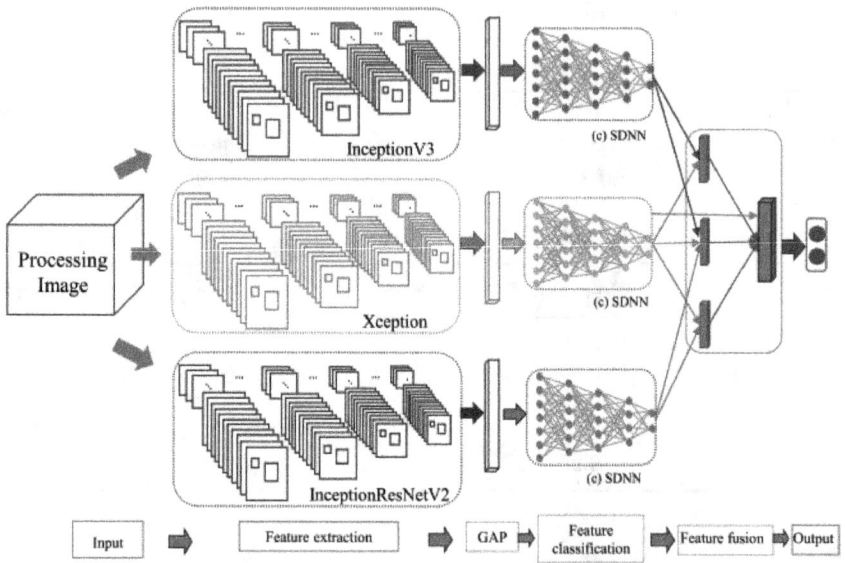

Fig. 5.5.   The structure of the neural networks for two-class classification.

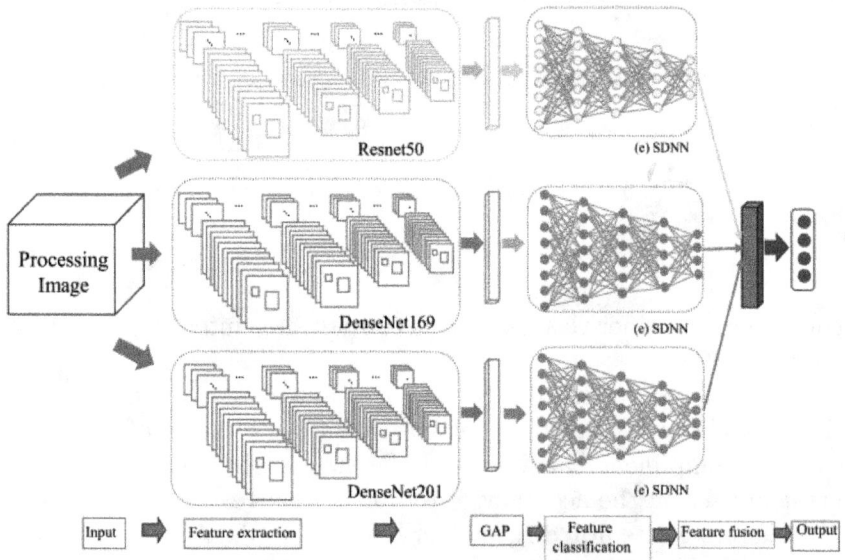

Fig. 5.6.   The structure of the neural networks for four-class classification.

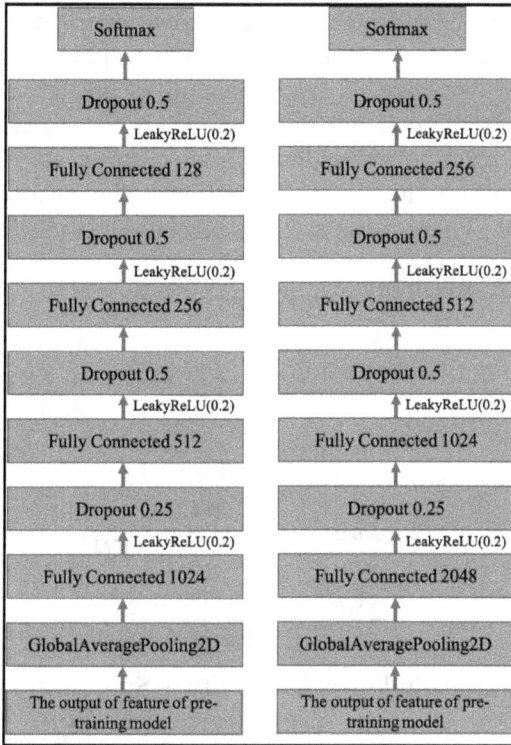

Fig. 5.7.   The SDNN blocks for two-class and four-class classification tasks.

5.4.3   *Metrics*

We utilized reliability and validity to evaluate the models and their ensembles. Reliability measures the degree of stability obtained by repeated tests under the same conditions. It can be assessed using the Kappa value. Kappa > 0.8 indicates excellent consistency. Validity reflects the degree of conformity between measured and actual values, as indicated by the following seven metrics.

Accuracy indicates the proportion of samples classified correctly. Precision is the proportion of positives correctly predicted. For early screening systems, sensitivity and specificity are important reference indicators of the referral decisions of screening options that directly indicate the effectiveness of the system. Sensitivity measures the proportion of positives correctly predicted, whereas specificity is the proportion of true negatives correctly identified as such. Given a typical balance between the two measures, a receiver operating characteristic curve with AUC can represent this balance graphically. The F1_score is the harmonic average of precision and recall. An F1_score score close to 1 indicates good performance. F_β is the weighted harmonic average of F1_score. As Youden's index approaches 1, the screening system exhibits enhanced authenticity; the reverse relationship is equally valid. These measures are presented in the following:

$$\text{Accuracy} = \frac{\text{TP} + \text{TN}}{\text{TP} + \text{FP} + \text{TN} + \text{FN}}, \tag{5.6}$$

$$\text{Sensitivity} = \frac{\text{TP}}{\text{TP+FN}}, \tag{5.7}$$

$$\text{Specificity} = \frac{\text{TN}}{\text{TN+FP}}, \tag{5.8}$$

$$\text{F1\_score} = \frac{2\text{TP}}{2\text{TP} + \text{FP} + \text{FN}}, \tag{5.9}$$

$$F_\beta = \frac{\left(1 + \beta^2\right) \times \text{Precision} \times \text{recall}}{\beta^2 \times \text{Precision} + \text{recall}}, \tag{5.10}$$

$$\text{Youden's index} = \text{Sensitivity} + \text{Specificity} - 1$$
$$= \frac{\text{TP} \times \text{TN} - \text{FN} \times \text{FP}}{(\text{TP+FN}) \times (\text{TN+FP})}. \tag{5.11}$$

where the samples can be divided into true positives (TP), false positives (FP), true negatives (TN), and false negatives (FN) in accordance with the combination of the real class and the classifier prediction category.

5.4.4 *Identification system*

The situation of classification imbalance was not serious. To reduce the computational cost, we selected three models (InceptionV3, InceptionResNetV2, and Xception) as alternative feature extractors, with ResNet50 as the baseline. These models largely represent the best learning abilities available. While making multiple combinations of these models, we expected the identification system to achieve the best performance.

After training these models independently (Fig. 5.8), we marked the models from strong to weak: Xception, InceptionV3, and

InceptionResNetV2 as 0, 1, and 2, respectively. First, the models were combined directly into an ensemble named Ens(012) by averaging their softmax scores. However, the performance did not match that of Xception. We speculated that the ideal number of component classifiers for binary classification problems may not simply be a result of the direct integration of the above three basic models. Thus, ensemble models consisting of two basic models were generated. The experiments showed that Ens(01) performed the best among all ensembles. We widen the ensemble models by combining these basic models with Ens(01) and Ens(02). Notably, Ens (0,01,02) exceeded well the previous best model Ens(01), and the result indicated that the optimal width of the ensemble may sometimes be useful. Therefore, the ensembles were further widened by combining the basic models with other ensemble models, such as Ens (0,2,02,01). The new results were almost better than those of Ens (012), but they were not as good as those of Ens (01). We replaced these basic models with the ones that performed well in the above experiments. Ens (0,01,02,012) showed a standout performance; hence, it was taken as the ensemble model of the task, for which it yielded the highest performance (Fig. 5.5). Figure 5.9 and Table 5.3 show the performance of the final ensemble. Table 5.5 presents the primary ensembles attempted and their performances under as many combinations as possible.

5.4.5   *Grading system*

5.4.5.1   *Two alternative strategies*

Regarding the grading system, we considered two alternative implementation strategies. The first strategy was a two-stage system: the first stage was a binary classification that distinguished between abnormal images and normal images via Xception, and the second stage was a ternary classification process to predict the level of DR severity on the basis of the abnormal data above via Resnet50. The alternative strategy was a quaternary classification model for predicting the level of DR severity on the basis of all testing images via Resnet50. The accuracy of the former was 94.1%, and the accuracy of the latter was 95.2%. The intuitive comparison (Fig. 5.10) showed that the strategy of the four-class classification worked the best.

Table 5.5.   Metrics of the identification system ensembles.

Model	Accuracy	Precision	Sensitivity	Specificity	Auc	Kappa	F1_score	F_β_score	Youden's Index
Xception[1]	0.9521	0.9491	0.9321	0.9782	0.9551	0.9032	0.9523	0.9503	0.9101
Baseline:Resnet 50	0.9342	0.9333	0.9332	0.9351	0.9342	0.9231	0.9322	0.9223	0.9223
0:Xception[2]	0.9715	0.9711	0.9740	0.9683	0.9712	0.9424	0.9715	0.9712	0.9424
1:InceptionV3	0.9676	0.9667	0.9622	0.9741	0.9682	0.9676	0.9669	0.9346	0.9363
2:IncepresV2[3]	0.9442	0.9435	0.9125	0.9828	0.9476	0.9444	0.9433	0.8883	0.8953
Ens(01)[4]	**0.9767**	0.9759	0.9716	**0.9828**	0.9772	0.9529	0.9767	0.9761	**0.9544**
Ens(02)[5]	0.9689	0.9677	0.9574	**0.9828**	0.9701	0.9373	0.9689	0.9680	0.9402
Ens(12)[6]	0.9598	0.9585	0.9456	0.9770	0.9613	0.9191	0.9599	0.9588	0.9226
3:Ens(012)[7]	0.9702	0.9691	0.9622	0.9799	0.9710	0.9340	0.9702	0.9694	0.9421
Ens(012,01)[8]	0.9689	0.9678	0.9598	0.9799	0.9698	0.9373	0.9689	0.9681	0.9397
Ens(012,02)[9]	0.9662	0.9652	0.9574	0.9770	0.9672	0.9321	0.9663	0.9655	0.9345
Ens(0,01,02)[10]	0.9753	0.9750	**0.9764**	0.9742	0.9752	0.9503	0.9753	0.9750	0.9505
Ens(0,2,01,02)[11]	0.9702	0.9691	0.9621	0.9799	0.9710	0.9399	0.9710	0.9694	0.9420
Ens(0,1,01,02)[12]	0.9740	0.9732	0.9693	0.9799	0.9746	0.9477	0.9741	0.9735	0.9492

Ens(0,01,02,3)[13]	**0.9767**	0.9760	0.9740	0.9799	0.9769	0.9529	0.9767	0.9762	0.9539
Ens(0,2,01,02,3)[14]	0.9701	0.9691	0.9622	0.9799	0.9710	0.9399	0.9702	0.9694	0.9421
Ens(0,1,01,02,3)[15]	0.9741	0.9732	0.9693	0.9799	0.9745	0.9477	0.9741	0.9735	0.9492
Ens (0,01,02,012)[16]	**0.9767**	**0.9760**	**0.9764**	**0.9800**	**0.9862**	**0.9530**	**0.9769**	**0.9762**	**0.9540**

Notes: [1]Xception: comparison of performances before preprocessing of Xception, [2]Xception: comparison of performances after preprocessing of Xception, [3]IncepresV2: InceptionResNetV2, [4]Ens(01): average of Xception and InceptionV3, [5]Ens(02): average of Xception and InceptionResNetV2, [6]Ens(12): average of InceptionV3 and InceptionResNetV2, [7]Ens(012): average of Xception, InceptionV3 and InceptionResV2, [8]Ens(012,01): average of Ens(012) and Ens(01), [9]Ens(012,02): average of Ens(012) and Ens(02), [10]Ens(0,02,02): average of Xception, Ens(02) and Ens(02), [11]Ens(0,2,02,12): average of Xception, InceptionResNetV2, Ens(02) and Ens(12), [12]Ens(0,1,01,02): average of Xception, InceptionV3, Ens(01),Ens(02) and Ens(012), [13]Ens(2,02,12,3): average of Xception, Ens(01),Ens(02) and Ens(012), [14]Ens(0,2,01,02,3): average of Xception, InceptionResNetV2, Ens(01), Ens(02), and Ens(012), [15]Ens(0,1,01,02,3): average of Xception, InceptionV3, Ens(01), Ens(02), and Ens(012), [16]Ens(0,01,02,012): average of Xception, Ens(01), Ens(02) and Ens(012).

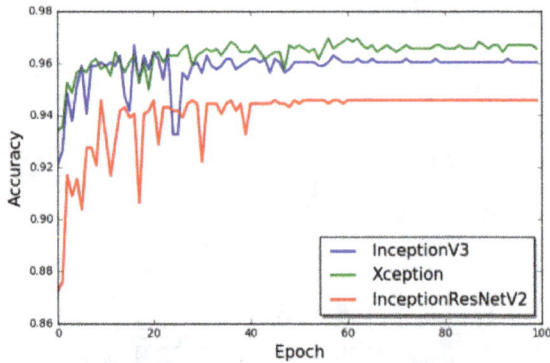

(a) Training accuracy curves

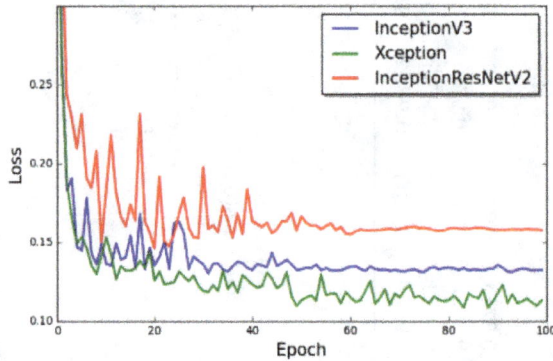

(b) Training loss curves

Fig. 5.8.   Training curves of the components of the identification system.

5.4.5.2   *Four-class classification*

The seven models discussed above were used in the experiments because of the thin granularity of multiple classification and the small amount of PDR data. The four-class experiments were divided into two groups by the models on the basis of their different input sizes (299×299, 224×224). From strong to weak, three models, i.e., InceptionV3, InceptionResNetV2, and Xception, were marked as 0, 1, and 2, respectively, in group one; the others, i.e., ResNet50, DenseNet169, DenseNet201, and DenseNet121, were marked as 4, 5, 6, and 7, respectively. First, we evaluated various ensembles in

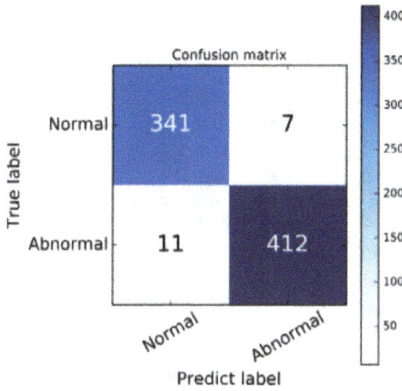

(a) Confusion matrix

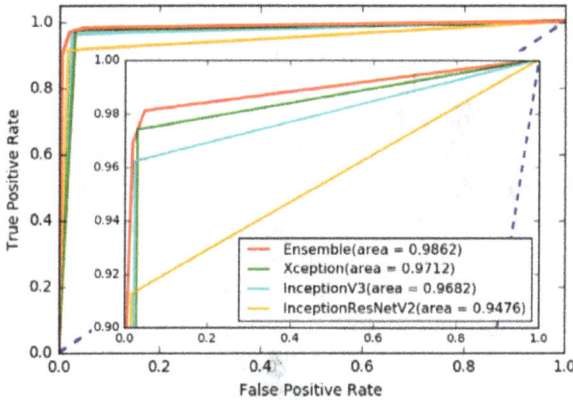

(b) ROC curves of components

Fig. 5.9. Confusion matrix and ROC curves of the identification system.

each group. Second, the outstanding models from the two groups were combined as much as possible to determine the final ensemble framework of the grading system.

Galton's theory states that combining many simple predictions is a force for accurate predictions. Hence, we combined all basic models directly. This step yielded Ens (0124567) with a remarkable accuracy rate of 96.36% relative to the other base learners above. Notably, the sensitivity and specificity of Ens (0124567) were 98.10% and 98.56%,

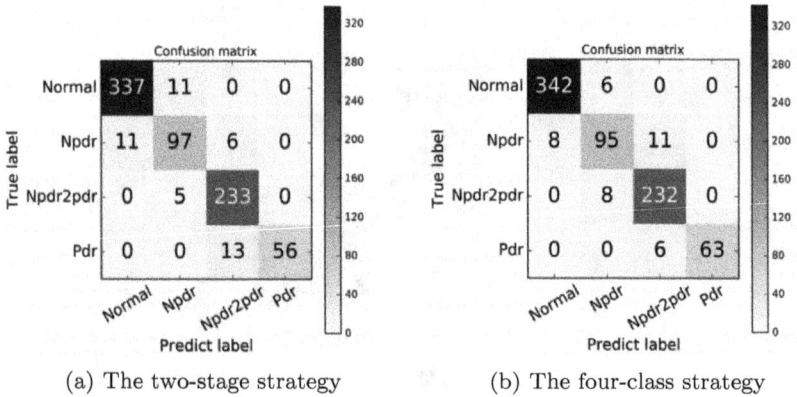

(a) The two-stage strategy (b) The four-class strategy

Fig. 5.10. Comparison of confusion matrices between two strategies of the Grading System.

respectively; however, it costs more than the pretrained models do. Inspired by the above binary experiments, we reduced the size of the ensembles to four. Moreover, the optimal number of component classifiers should be similar to the number of class labels in some studies (Hernández-Lobato *et al.*, 2013; Bonab and Can, 2016, 2019). The results showed that Ens (4567) had a high accuracy of 96.23% under the condition involving the same number of base learners. Sequentially, we reduced the size of the ensembles to three. The top three single models (0,4,5) were integrated into Ens (045); however, its accuracy was only 94.94%. Subsequently, we replaced the third-ranked model 2: InceptionV3 with the fourth-ranked model 5: DenseNet201; this step yielded Ens (456) with an accuracy of 96.50% and other relatively high indicators. A variety of integrations were further attempted, and similar performances were achieved; however, the results did not exceed the current level. Therefore, our judgment was correct. In other words, an optimal number of component classifiers exists and might be near the number of class tags with subtle adjustments depending on the specific task. Figure 5.5 shows the Ens (456) framework, and Fig. 5.11 shows its performance. Further information about the evaluation metrics is shown in Tables 5.6–5.8.

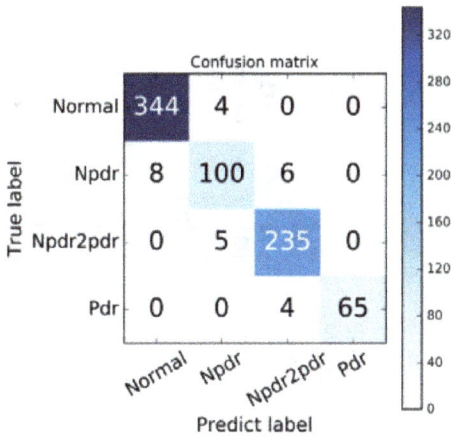

(a) Confusion matrix

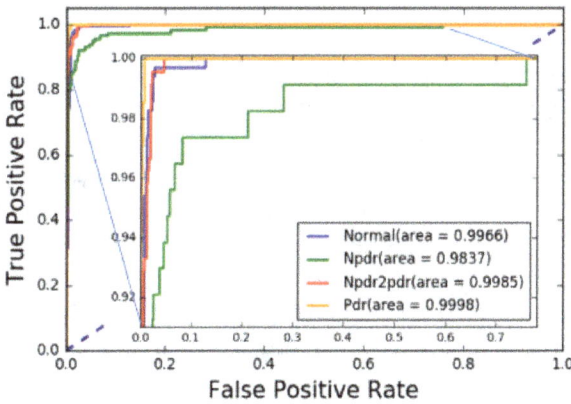

(b) ROC curves

Fig. 5.11.   Confusion matrix and ROC curves of the grading system.

5.4.6   *Analysis of experiments*

The UK National Institute for Clinical Excellence guidelines state that a DR screening test should have at least a sensitivity of 80% and a specificity of 95%. In our work, the identification model performed

Table 5.6.　Metrics of the grading system ensembles: the first group, the input is (299 × 299).

Model	Accuracy	Recall	Precision	Sensitivity	Specificity	Kappa	F1_score	F_β_score	Youden's index
0: InceptionV3	0.9455	0.9260	0.9376	0.9787	0.9655	0.8811	0.9449	0.9349	0.9442
1: IncepresV2	0.9416	0.9072	0.9072	0.9764	0.9741	0.9123	0.9410	0.9306	0.9505
2: Xception	0.9209	0.8809	0.9001	0.9622	0.9828	0.8811	0.9201	0.9959	0.9449
Ens(01)[1]	0.9442	0.9101	0.9408	0.9788	0.9770	0.9436	0.9436	0.9336	0.9460
Ens(01)$_m$	0.9442	0.9101	0.9408	0.9788	0.9770	0.9162	0.9436	0.9336	0.9557
Ens(02)[2]	0.9507	0.9332	0.9431	0.9811	0.9684	0.9262	0.9503	0.9409	0.9495
Ens(02)$_m$	0.9468	0.9267	0.9396	0.9787	0.9684	0.9203	0.9461	0.9367	0.9471
Ens(12)[3]	0.9429	0.9094	0.9387	0.9787	0.9741	0.9143	0.9424	0.9318	0.9529
Ens(12)$_m$	0.9416	0.9072	0.9377	0.9764	0.9741	0.9123	0.9411	0.9306	0.9505
3: Ens(012)[4]	0.9520	0.9701	0.9677	0.9811	0.9770	0.9280	0.9517	0.9423	0.9581
Ens(012)$_m$	0.9442	0.9101	0.9408	0.9787	0.9770	0.9162	0.9436	0.9336	0.9557
Ens(3,0)[5]	0.9455	0.9262	0.9377	0.9787	0.9626	0.9184	0.9449	0.9350	0.9414
Ens(3,1)[6]	0.9416	0.9072	0.9376	0.9764	0.9741	0.9123	0.9410	0.9306	0.9505
Ens(3,2)[7]	0.9494	0.9217	0.9406	0.9764	0.9770	0.9241	0.9489	0.9365	0.9534
Ens(3,2)$_m$	0.9416	0.9072	0.9377	0.9764	0.9741	0.9123	0.9410	0.9306	0.9505
Ens(3,01)[8]	**0.9546**	**0.9282**	**0.9529**	**0.9811**	**0.9799**	**0.9318**	**0.9542**	**0.9473**	**0.9610**
Ens(3,01)$_m$	0.9533	0.9260	0.9518	0.9810	0.9799	0.9299	0.9528	0.9459	0.9610
Ens(3,02)[9]	0.9494	0.9281	0.9432	0.9787	0.9713	0.9242	0.9488	0.9398	0.9500
Ens(3,02)$_m$	0.9494	0.9296	0.9423	0.9787	0.9684	0.9242	0.9490	0.9396	0.9471

Ens(01,02)[10]	0.9494	0.9310	0.9421	0.9787	0.9684	0.9242	0.9489	0.9396	0.9471
Ens(01, 02)$_m$	0.9520	0.9324	0.9463	0.9787	0.9741	0.9281	0.9513	0.9432	0.9529
Ens(3,Ens(01, 02)$_m$)[11]	0.9533	0.9306	0.9489	0.9787	0.9741	0.9300	0.9528	0.9449	0.9529
Ens(3, Ens(01, 02)$_m$)$_m$	0.9520	0.9310	0.9465	0.9787	0.9741	0.9280	0.9515	0.9431	0.9529

Notes: [1]Ens(01): average of InceptionV3 and IncepresV2; Ens(01)$_m$: max of them, [2]Ens(02): average of InceptionV3 and Xception; ; Ens(02)$_m$ = max of them, [3]Ens(12): average of InceptionV3, IncepresV2 and Xception; Ens(12)$_m$ = max of them, [4]Ens(012): average of IncepresV2 and Xception; Ens(012)$_m$ = max of them, [5]Ens(3,0): average (max) of Ens(012) and InceptionV3, [6]Ens(3,1): average (max) or max of Ens(012) and IncepresV2, [7]Ens(3,2): average of Ens(012) and Xception; Ens(3,2)$_m$ = max of them, [8]Ens(3,01): average of Ens(012) and Ens(01); Ens(3,01)$_m$ = max of them, [9]Ens(3,02): average of Ens(012) and Ens(02); Ens(3,02)$_m$ = average of Ens(012) and Ens(02); Ens(3,02)$_m$ = max of them, [10]Ens(01,02): average of Ens(01) and Ens(02); Ens(01,02)$_m$ = max of them, [11]Ens(3,Ens(01,02)$_m$): average of Ens(012), Ens(01,02)$_m$; Ens(3, Ens(01,02)$_m$)$_m$ = max of them.

Table 5.7.   Metrics of the grading system ensembles: The second group, the input is (224 × 224).

Model	Accuracy	Recall	Precision	Sensitivity	Specificity	Kappa	F1_score	F_β_score	Youden's index
4: Resnet50	0.9494	0.9240	0.9451	0.9811	0.9828	0.9241	0.9491	0.9404	0.9638
5: DN_169	0.9469	0.9195	0.9466	0.9551	0.9914	0.9199	0.9464	0.9406	0.9465
6: DN_201	0.9429	0.9140	0.9333	0.9811	0.9741	0.9144	0.9421	0.9289	0.9552
7: DN_121	0.9364	0.9162	0.9222	0.9740	0.9741	0.9052	0.9372	0.9203	0.9481
Ens(45)[1]	0.9507	0.9261	0.9463	0.9811	0.9828	0.9261	0.9504	0.9418	0.9638
Ens(46)[2]	0.9546	0.9295	0.9534	0.9811	0.9828	0.9318	0.9540	0.9480	0.9638
Ens(47)[3]	0.9507	0.9273	0.9456	0.9811	0.9826	0.9261	0.9506	0.9415	0.9638
Ens(56)[4]	0.9494	0.9190	0.9450	0.9787	0.9856	0.9239	0.9485	0.9390	0.9644
Ens(57)[5]	0.9494	0.9241	0.9450	0.9645	0.9885	0.9240	0.9491	0.9403	0.9530
Ens(67)[6]	0.9481	0.9186	0.9428	0.9787	0.9798	0.9220	0.9472	0.9373	0.9586
8:Ens(456)[7]	**0.9650**	**0.9467**	**0.9635**	0.9811	0.9885	**0.9475**	**0.9647**	**0.9599**	**0.9696**
Ens(456)$_m$	0.9546	0.9295	0.9534	0.9811	0.9828	0.9318	0.9540	0.9480	0.9638
Ens(457)[8]	0.9571	0.9319	0.9561	0.9787	0.9885	0.9357	0.9567	0.9508	0.9508

Ens(467)[9]	0.9611	0.9402	0.9572	0.9834	0.9828	0.9417	0.9610	0.9535	0.9662
Ens(567)[10]	0.9611	0.9347	0.9589	0.9764	0.9914	0.9415	0.9605	0.9535	0.9508
9:Ens(4567)[11]	0.9623	0.9412	0.9616	0.9787	0.9856	0.9435	0.9620	0.9572	0.9644
Ens(4567)$_m$	0.9546	0.9295	0.9534	0.9811	0.9828	0.9318	0.9540	0.9480	0.9638
Ens(8,9,467)[12]	0.9611	0.9405	0.9595	0.9787	0.9828	0.9416	0.9609	0.9554	0.9615
Ens(8,9,567)[13]	0.9637	0.9434	0.9639	0.9763	0.9885	0.9454	0.9632	0.9594	0.9649
Ens(7,56,9,567)[14]	0.9650	0.9387	0.9635	0.9764	**0.9913**	0.9473	0.9645	0.9580	0.9678

Notes: [1]Ens(45): average of Resnet50 and DN_169, [2]Ens(46): average of Resnet50 and DN_201, [3]Ens(47): average of Resnet50 and DN_121, [4]Ens(56): average of DN_169 and DN_201, [5]Ens(57): average of DN_169 and DN_121, [6]Ens(67): average of DN_201 and DN_121, [7]Ens(456): average of Resnet50,DN_169 and DN_201; Ens(456)$_m$: max of them, [8]Ens(457): average of Resnet50,DN_169 and DN_121, [9]Ens(467): average of Resnet50,DN_201 and DN_121, [10]Ens(567): average of DN_169,DN_201 and DN_121, [11]Ens(4567): average of Resnet50,DN_169,DN_201 and DN_121; Ens(4567)$_m$: max of them, [12]Ens(456,8,467): average of Ens(456),Ens(4567),Ens(467), [13]Ens(456,8,567): average of Ens(456),Ens(4567),Ens(567), [14]Ens(7,56,8,567): average of DN_121,Ens(56),Ens(4567) and Ens(567).

well with a sensitivity of 97.5%, a specificity of 97.7%, and an accuracy of 97.7%. By contrast, the grading model achieved a sensitivity of 98.1%, a specificity of 98.9%, and an accuracy of 96.5%. Therefore, the models achieved satisfactory performance on our dataset.

From the experiments, we found that the stronger the base learner was, the higher the performance was generally; moreover, the effects of the ensembles with multiple-ensemble classifiers were stronger than those of the dull ensemble models in some cases. We noted that some results degenerated after the ensemble phase in the four-class experiments. We conjectured this degeneration was primarily caused by the model selection strategy in the ensemble phase: various base learners of different depths can implicitly learn different levels of semantic image representation. On the basis of model complementarity, the posterior probabilities of these weak learners can be fused to predict the modalities of unseen images. Compared with the max method in Table 5.6, the averaging method was effective in our work because it reduced the variances of the components substantively (Ju *et al.*, 2018; Szegedy *et al.*, 2015).

5.5   Discussion

During the design of the two ensemble models, we made several considerations in the following aspects.

(1) **Combined strategy of components:** The frameworks of the two classification tasks searched for the ideal combination of component classifiers on the basis of the number of class tags in the dataset as a guide. We assumed that the basic components used in our experiments were all independent. In the experiments, we found that arbitrarily increasing or decreasing the number of component classifiers would reduce the performance of the model. Moreover, different combinations of methods of the component classifiers were important in achieving the best integration performance. However, the diversity of the real-world dataset, the complexity of the task, and the degree of independence of existing component classifiers under the constraint of computational resource requirements did not guarantee this assumption in most cases; thus, determining the integration framework of a given set classifier on real data remains a challenging problem.

(2) **Model optimization:** In view of the limited dataset and the deep models used in the system, we should note the problem of gradient disappearance. On the basis of the unsupervised layer-wise training (Bengio *et al.*, 2007), we proposed a supervised block-wise training strategy. Each SDNN of a component classifier was briefly used as an independent model, and it was trained with high-level features as input via the corresponding pretrained feature extractor model. After the SDNN was separately trained, it could be connected to the corresponding feature extractor to form a component classifier; the feature extractor module could be initialized with the pretrained weight, and the optimal weight obtained after the SDNN independent training could be used as its pretrained weight to initialize itself. Subsequently, the entire component classifier could be trained using fine-tuning after the training. This training arrangement increased the speed of the convergence of the whole classification component. In sum, the entire component was divided into several blocks for training; a good setting of weight parameters was found for each block, and the component was then globally optimized in accordance with the local optimal weight of each block while minimizing the training cost.

(3) **Several obvious advantages:** First, the reproducibility and consistency of diagnostic results could provide clinicians with insights into the diagnostic process. Additionally, the two different systems could be used to match different application requirements. When screening populations with substantial diseases, achieving high sensitivity and high specificity is critical to minimize false-positive and false-negative results. Finally, a quick reporting of auxiliary diagnostic results could improve clinicians' efficiency.

(4) **Some limitations:** The annotation work was based on the clinical experience of the ophthalmologist graders. Therefore, the algorithm may perform differently when used in images with subtle findings that a majority of clinicians could not identify. Another fundamental limitation arises from the black box, which is the nature of deep networks. The network automatically learns the features from the images and associated grade; however, the specific features by which the networks are formed are unknown. Understanding the aspects used by deep neural networks to make predictions is an active area of research.

In the future, a large training dataset containing tens of thousands of abnormal cases must be collected from other hospitals via various types of cameras to improve the models' generalization. Second, the visualization of the aspects learned by CNNs is important as it can improve the interpretability of diagnostic results by identifying the source regions of features associated with a specified classification result, as well as the magnitude of the feature intensity. Additionally, doctors can make an accurate diagnosis on the basis of visualization results. Third, in the case of a medical dataset of limited scale, further discussing the design and research of ensemble frameworks from a theoretical perspective is necessary.

5.6 DeepDR: An AI System for DR Diagnosis

In order to facilitate the use of our model in the clinical environment, we built an intelligent DR detection system named DeepDR. The DeepDR deployed the trained model in the cloud and provided services to the hospital through the Internet. As shown in Fig. 5.12, the DeepDR mainly includes the following basic components:

(1) **The web server:** The web server is the main operation component of DeepDR. Its main functions include providing the operation such as managing and operating patients' data, calling the discrimination and diagnosis services provided by the model server, and generating diagnosis reports.

(2) **Database server:** The database server is the storage component of the DeepDR. It is mainly responsible for storing and maintaining users' information, diagnosis records, operation logs, and other system usage information.

(3) **Model server:** The model server is a diagnostic component of the DeepDR. In addition to providing DR grading service for fundus images, it also provides image quality judgment, left and right eye discrimination for fundus images, and other services.

When applying the DeepDR as an AI-aided diagnosis system, the doctor first logs into the system through the browser and uploads the patient's fundus images collected by the fundus camera to the

Table 5.8. Metrics of the Grading system Ensembles: Integration.

Model	Accuracy	Recall	Precision	Sensitivity	Specificity	Kappa	F1_score	F_β_score	Youden's index
Ens(04)[1]	0.9559	0.9292	0.9716	0.9828	0.9885	0.9336	0.9552	0.9506	0.9544
Ens(045)[2]	0.9494	0.9242	0.9448	0.9645	0.9885	0.9240	0.9491	0.9403	0.9530
Ens(0456)[3]	0.9494	0.9242	0.9448	0.9645	0.9885	0.9240	0.9491	0.9403	0.9530
10:Ens(0124567)[4]	0.9637	0.9411	0.9647	0.9810	0.9856	0.9454	0.9632	0.9594	0.9667
Ens(01567)[5]	0.9624	0.9404	0.9634	0.9812	0.9856	0.9435	0.9618	0.9582	0.9667
Ens(01,56)[6]	0.9624	0.9406	0.9632	0.9811	0.9856	0.9435	0.9615	0.9577	0.9667
Ens(8,10)[7]	0.9624	0.9406	0.9632	0.9811	0.9856	0.9435	0.9615	0.9577	0.9667
Ens(Ens(3,01),8,10)[8]	0.9611	0.9353	0.9627	0.9811	0.9856	0.9414	0.9605	0.9564	0.9667
Ens(3,9,567)[9]	0.9611	0.9353	0.9627	0.9811	0.9856	0.9414	0.9605	0.9564	0.9667
Ens(Ens(3,01),9,567)[10]	0.9637	0.9412	0.9644	0.9834	0.9856	0.9454	0.9632	0.9564	0.9690
Ens(9,567)	0.9611	0.9428	0.9584	0.9787	0.9856	0.9416	0.9608	0.9550	0.9644

Notes: [1]Ens(04): average of InceptionV3 and Resnet50, [2]Ens(045): average of InceptionV3 and Resnet50, [3]Ens(0456): average of InceptionV3, Resnet50,DN_169, [4]Ens(0124567): average of all models, [5]Ens(01567): average of InceptionV3, Resnet50,DN_169,and DN_201, [6]Ens(01,56): average of Ens(01) and Ens(56), [7]Ens(8,10): average of **Ens(456)** and InceptionV3Resnet50,DN_169,and DN_201, [8]Ens(Ens(3,01),8,10): average of Ens(3,01),Ens(456) and Ens(01567), [9]Ens(3,8,567): average of Ens(012),Ens(4567) and Ens(567), [10]Ens(Ens(3,01),9,567): average of Ens(012),Ens(4567) and Ens(567).

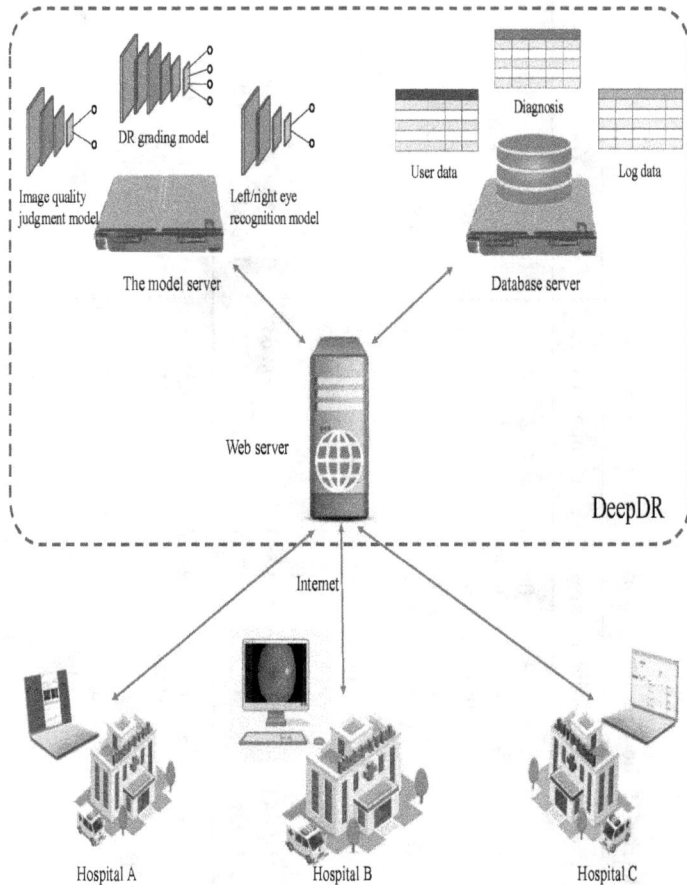

Fig. 5.12.   The architecture of the DeepDR.

web server in the form of a folder for each patient. After receiving the fundus images, the web server first applies a model to judge the image quality to detect the non-fundus images and the unqualified fundus images. The unqualified images' information is fed back to the user through the browser. If the fundus images are qualified, the web server will call an AI model to distinguish the left and right eyes of the images. Then, the web server will establish left and right eye image folders for each patient and call the DR diagnosis model to diagnose the left and right eyes of the patient. After the diagnosis is completed, the user can view the diagnosis results given by the system on the page and can choose to print the diagnosis results as a formal diagnosis report.

We verified the performance of the model in the clinical environment by trials in various hospitals. The medical personnel upload the collected fundus color photos to the system, and the model makes decision on the images and returns the results to the user. At the same time, in the backend of the website, the ophthalmologist team manually annotated the uploaded images and compared them with the results of model diagnosis. Finally, for 259 out of 282 qualified data, the model's results were the same as those annotated by the ophthalmologist. The consistency reached 91.8%, which indicates that our model also has good adaptability for clinical application.

5.7   Conclusion

In conclusion, a high-quality labeled medical imaging DR dataset was built, and an identification and grading system of DR called DeepDR was proposed. The relationship between the number of ideal component classifiers and the number of class labels was verified and explored. Using nine medical metrics, we evaluated the models in terms of validity and reliability. The results demonstrated that DeepDR worked satisfactorily.

Furthermore, we, together with the ophthalmologist team of Sichuan Provincial People's Hospital, constructed a moderate-scale and well-annotated DR dataset. On the basis of this dataset, we built a deep convolution neural network model for the characteristics of DR. We further built an intelligent system named DeepDR and deployed our model in the cloud to provide online diagnosis services for ophthalmologists. The validation in the laboratory and in the actual clinical applications shows that our model has reached a high accuracy and has good clinical significance.

Chapter 6

Automated Segmentation of Macular Edema in OCT Using Deep Neural Networks

Macular edema is an eye disease that can affect visual acuity. Typical disease symptoms include subretinal fluid (SRF) and pigment epithelium detachment (PED). Optical coherence tomography (OCT) has been widely used for diagnosing macular edema because of its non-invasive and high-resolution properties. Segmentation for macular edema lesions from OCT images plays an important role in clinical diagnosis. Many computer-aided systems have been proposed for the segmentation. Most traditional segmentation methods used in these systems are based on low-level handcrafted features which require significant domain knowledge and are sensitive to the variations of lesions. To overcome these shortcomings, this paper proposes to use deep neural networks (DNNs) together with atrous spatial pyramid pooling (ASPP) to automatically segment the SRF and PED lesions. Lesion-related features are first extracted by DNNs and then processed by ASPP which is composed of multiple atrous convolutions with different fields of view to accommodate the various scales of the lesions. Based on ASPP, a novel module called stochastic ASPP (sASPP) is proposed to combat the co-adaptation of multiple atrous convolutions. A large OCT dataset provided by a competition platform called "AI Challenger" is used to train and evaluate the proposed model. Experimental results demonstrate that the DNNs together with ASPP achieve higher segmentation accuracy compared with the state-of-the-art method. The stochastic operation added in sASPP is empirically verified as an effective regularization method that can alleviate the overfitting problem and significantly reduce the validation error.

6.1 Introduction

The macula is located in the central part of the retina and is the main sensory region for detecting light signals. Impairment of the macula impacts visual acuity to varying degrees. Macular edema, character-ized by an accumulation of fluid near the fovea in the macula, is a common reason for vision loss (Goatman, 2006). Macular edema does not signify a particular ocular disease but a series of macular responses to retinal environment alternation (Coscas *et al.*, 2010), including pigment epithelium detachment (PED) and subretinal fluid (SRF). Common causes of macular edema include age-related macu-lar degeneration, diabetic retinopathy, and intraocular surgery. Early diagnosis and timely treatment of macular edema can help reduce vision loss.

Optical coherence tomography (OCT) is a non-invasive imaging technology introduced in 1991 that has been widely used in the clinical evaluation of macular edema (Huang *et al.*, 1991; Coscas *et al.*, 2010; Tranos *et al.*, 2004). Compared with other imaging modalities such as fluorescein angiography, the advantages of OCT include its non-invasive property, rapid imaging, high reproducibil-ity, and safety profile (Trichonas and Kaiser, 2014). OCT is based on the interferometric principle that generates cross-sectional images in high resolution. It can delineate multiple retinal layers and visualize the structural changes of the retina in large areas (Wolf and Wolf-Schnurrbusch, 2010). The A scan (one dimension) in depth is recon-structed using the reflective signal, and a number of A scans are used to construct the B scan slice (two dimensions) (Drexler *et al.*, 2003). The complete OCT volume is composed of multiple B scan slices. In the OCT slices, normal and abnormal tissues have a different appear-ance because of their distinct reflectivity patterns. Figure 6.1 shows four slices, which represent the appearance of normal and abnormal tissues.

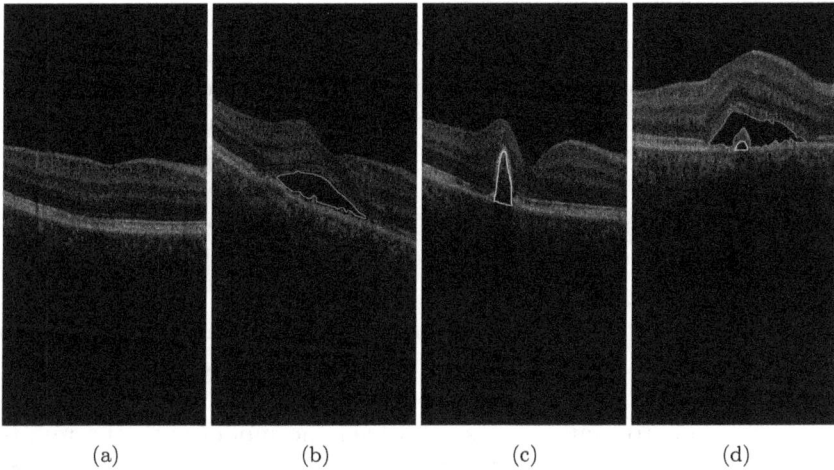

(a)   (b)   (c)   (d)

Fig. 6.1. Appearance of normal and macular edema tissues in OCT. The lesions of SRF and PED are marked by red and green, respectively.

The accurate segmentation of macular edema-related lesions is required for quantification in clinical practice. However, the manual annotation of lesions is subjective, labor-intensive, and prone to errors. This is mainly caused by the limited use of prior knowledge about the distorted morphology and the blurred boundaries near the lesions (Xu *et al.*, 2017). Many computer-aided systems have been proposed to assist ophthalmologists in the clinical diagnosis of macular edema. Conventional segmentation methods in these systems include threshold-based and graph-based approaches that use handcrafted features (Chen *et al.*, 2013; Penha *et al.*, 2012; Ahlers *et al.*, 2008). However, these low-level features are sensitive to image quality and require significant domain knowledge. In this paper, we aim to automatically segment SRF and PED lesions in OCT images using deep neural networks (DNNs). Different from conventional methods that use elaborate handcrafted features, DNNs learn to extract different levels of features from low to high as the depth of the network increases. Many novel networks have been proposed to perform segmentation tasks, including FCN (Long *et al.*, 2015), UNet (Ronneberger *et al.*, 2015), SegNet (Badrinarayanan *et al.*, 2017), and DeepLab (Chen *et al.*, 2017). Based on these networks, some studies have been conducted to segment macular edema-related lesions in an end-to-end manner. Significantly, ReLayNet (Roy *et al.*, 2017) and 3D U-Net (De Fauw *et al.*, 2018), which are DNN-based methods, have achieved better performance in fluid segmentation task compared with traditional methods. These results demonstrate that DNNs are promising approaches in macular edema segmentation tasks.

Although DNN-based models have achieved remarkable performance in macular edema segmentation tasks, the depth of neural networks in current studies is relatively shallow. For example, the encoder and decoder parts in ReLayNet are both networks with six layers. The question is whether the depth of the model could help improve segmentation accuracy. Moreover, macular edema-related lesions typically have multiple scales from small to large. The conventional method to manage this is to feed the model with the inputs rescaled multiple times and then aggregate the features. However, this approach has a high computational cost. Based on the above considerations, in this paper, DNN with a considerably greater depth [e.g., ResNet50 (He *et al.*, 2016a)] is used as an encoder to extract highly abstract features from the OCT image. Then, atrous spatial pyramid pooling (ASPP) (Chen *et al.*, 2017), which has been successfully applied to the semantic image segmentation task, is used to process these features. ASPP is based on atrous convolution (Chen *et al.*, 2017), which is a special convolution operation with "holes" inserted between the elements of the kernel. Atrous convolution can effectively increase the field of view of the kernel but does not incur more learnable parameters and computational cost. ASPP works by using multiple atrous convolutions with different fields of view to capture features at multiple scales. In the experimental section, we empirically demonstrate that ASPP together with features from ResNet50 has better segmentation accuracy than ReLeyNet and U-Net.

Based on ASPP, a novel module that combines atrous convolution and randomness is proposed in this paper. The proposed module is called stochastic ASPP (sASPP) because features from atrous convolutions in ASPP may be randomly dropped (or retained) during the training phase. An example of sASPP in the encoder–decoder segmentation model is presented in Fig. 6.2. The input of sASPP is the highly abstract feature from the DNN-based encoder network

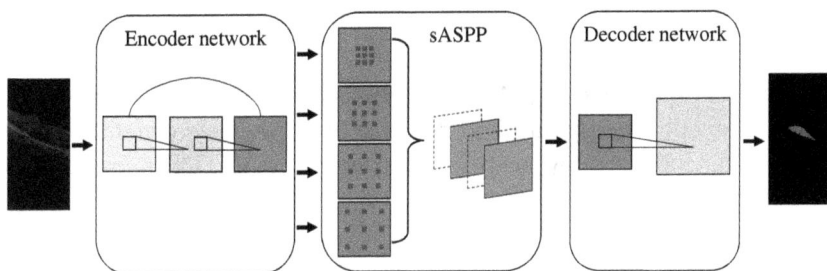

Fig. 6.2. Proposed sASPP in the encoder–decoder-based segmentation model. The dashed line denotes that the feature maps are dropped during training.

and is independently processed by the atrous convolutions. The main difference between ASPP and sASPP is the random drop operation applied to the feature maps produced by the atrous convolutions. In this example, there are two feature maps dropped (indicated by the dashed line). sASPP is proposed to prevent the co-adaptation of the atrous convolutions in ASPP. Moreover, the proposed sASPP can be regarded as 2^n possible models, suppose there are n atrous convolutions. The proposed sASPP should have better performance compared with ASPP because the latter uses the multiple atrous convolutions statically, whereas sASPP attempts to use a number of possible combinations of them. The experimental results demonstrate that the proposed sASPP is an effective regularization method that achieves lower errors on the validation dataset. The main contributions of this study are summarized as follows:

(i) ASPP together with an encoder–decoder model is used to segment the SRF and PED lesions in OCT images. The method has superior accuracy compared with the state-of-the-art method.

(ii) A module called sASPP is further proposed, which stochastically drops the feature maps from the atrous convolutions in ASPP. Randomness in sASPP is assumed to prevent the co-adaptation of the atrous convolutions.

(iii) The experimental results demonstrate that sASPP is an effective regularization method to alleviate the overfitting problem. Compared with ASPP, the proposed sASPP can achieve higher segmentation accuracy while maintaining lower errors on the validation dataset.

6.2   Related Works

In this section, an overview of previous studies based on the traditional graph theory method for macular edema segmentation is presented, followed by a brief introduction of DNNs and their applications.

6.2.1   *Traditional methods for segmenting macular edema*

Graph theory has been widely used to segment anatomical and pathological structures in OCT images (Haeker *et al.*, 2007; Garvin *et al.*, 2009; Chiu *et al.*, 2010, 2015). Each OCT slice image can be considered as a graph, where each pixel corresponds to a node in the graph. Nodes are connected by edges with assigned weights. The task is to travel across the graph from a start node to an end node with the minimum sum of weights. Then, the preferred pathway is the boundary between the pathological and normal structures in the segmentation task. The appropriate weight assignment to the edge and the solution of the minimum sum of weights between two nodes are the two keys in graph-based method. Particularly, the intensity gradients are used to estimate the weights, followed by Dijkstra's algorithm to determine the lowest weighted path of the graph in Chiu *et al.* (2010) to segment the retinal layers. This method was further improved by a subsequent study that applied constraints to add prior information (Dufour *et al.*, 2012). Moreover, Chiu *et al.* (2015) proposed segmenting the retinal layers together with the fluid regions using a two-stage segmentation method. In the first stage, the kernel regression method is used to generate coarse segmentation results. Graph theory is then used to refine the boundaries in the second stage.

In addition to the aforementioned graph-based method, there also exist other machine learning-based methods, such as k-nearest neighbor (k-NN) (Chen *et al.*, 2012) and random forest (Lang *et al.*, 2015). These traditional methods have achieved progress in the retinal layer or fluid segmentation task; however, some limitations should be noted. First, these methods depend heavily on handcrafted, low-level features, which have limited representation ability and are sensitive to image quality. Second, the traditional methods typically divide the segmentation procedure into several stages, and the errors in the previous stage may be amplified in the latter stages. Moreover, significant domain knowledge is required in the designation of hand-crafted features and segmentation stages. These potential limitations have constrained the wide application of conventional segmentation methods in the clinical analysis of macular edema.

6.2.2   *Deep neural networks for segmenting macular edema*

DNNs are composed of multiple layers that transform the input non-linearly layer by layer in a data-driven manner. Two types of neural networks, that is, feed forward neural networks (FNNs) (LeCun *et al.*, 1998; He *et al.*, 2016b) and recurrent neural networks (RNNs) (Williams and Zipser, 1989; Yi and Tan, 2004; Yi, 2010), have been heavily studied during the recent decades. Since 2012 when AlexNet (Krizhevsky *et al.*, 2012) won the ILSVRC-2012 competition, there have been revolutionary advances in computer vision tasks using DNNs. These achievements can be attributed to several factors, including novel network architecture, graphics processing units (GPUs) with powerful computation ability, and large-scale annotated dataset. In addition to computer vision tasks, DNNs have been successfully applied to medical image analysis applications, such as retinopathy of prematurity (Hu *et al.*, 2018), lymph node (Anthimopoulos *et al.*, 2016), and breast cancer classification tasks (Carneiro *et al.*, 2017).

A recent study that used a U-Net-based network called ReLayNet (Roy *et al.*, 2017) was the first work to use fully convolutional neural networks in retinal layer and fluid segmentation tasks. ReLayNet is composed of two parts, an encoder and a decoder, both of which are based on neural networks with six layers. The encoder network is constructed by convolutional and pooling layers in turn, which are designed to extract features from the input OCT image. The decoder network attempts to predict the category of each raw pixel by processing features from the encoder network using alternating convolutional and unpooling layers. The unpooling layer upsamples the features using the indices from the corresponding pooling layer, which helps accurately segment the fluid with small regions. The upsampled features are then concatenated with those from the encoder network that have an identical spatial size. ReLayNet is trained end-to-end and has demonstrated superior performance compared with conventional segmentation methods. Besides ReLayNet, a 3D U-Net network (De Fauw *et al.*, 2018) is also used to segment the lesions in OCT images. Based on the segmentation results produced by the 3D U-Net, classification networks are further used to give diagnoses and referrals. The two-stage framework can reduce the error caused by data from different devices.

The depth of neural networks is a critical factor, where the network with deep depth probes extracts features with a high abstraction level. However, one major limitation of ReLayNet and 3D U-Net is the comparatively shallow depth in the encoder, which may impede segmentation performance. In this paper, a novel module called sASPP is proposed to accurately segment macular edema-related lesions. sASPP is based on ASPP, which is a module composed of multiple atrous convolutions with different fields of view, whereas sASPP stochastically drops features from each atrous convolution. sASPP has three advantages over ReLayNet. First, the input of sASPP is from a very deep neural network (e.g., ResNet50), which can discriminatively represent the data. Second, the multiple atrous convolutions with different fields of view in sASPP can adapt to objects of various scales. Third, the randomness in sASPP helps alleviate the overfitting problem in the segmentation task.

6.3   Methodology

In this section, the ASPP is introduced, including the definition of atrous convolution and features in multiple scales. Then, the proposed ASPP with randomness is illustrated in detail.

6.3.1   *Atrous spatial pyramid pooling*

6.3.1.1   *Atrous convolution*

In the convolution operation, the parameters are kernels that connect with the input locally. An example of a convolution operation is

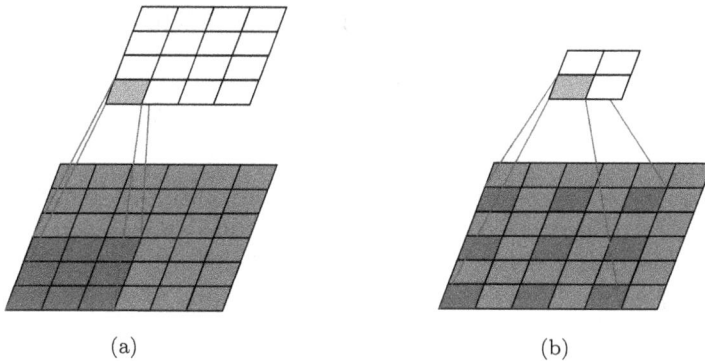

(a)   (b)

Fig. 6.3. Comparison between convolution and atrous convolution operations. (a) Convolution operation for which the kernel size is 3 and stride is 1. (b) Atrous convolution operation for which the kernel size is 3, stride is 1, and rate is 2. Both kernels in the two types of operations are shared among each location in the inputs.

shown in Fig. 6.3(a). The convolution operation can be formulated as

$$z_{v,u}^{l+1} = \sum_{c=0}^{C^l-1} \sum_{p=0}^{P^l-1} \sum_{q=0}^{Q^l-1} a_{v+p,u+q,c}^l \cdot w_{p,q,c}^l, \tag{6.1}$$

where P, Q, and C denote the dimensions of the convolution kernel and their corresponding lower-case letters denote the cursor in kernel w^l. $z_{v,u}^{l+1}$ denotes the input of location (v, u) in the $l+1$ layer, which is computed by the convolution operation of kernel w^l and the previous layer's output a^l. $a_{v,u}^{l+1}$ can be computed by applying nonlinear transformations [e.g., batch normalization (Ioffe and Szegedy, 2015) and ReLU (Glorot *et al.*, 2011)] to $z_{v,u}^{l+1}$. Typically, convolution operations in modern networks often have small kernels, such as 3×3. Increasing the field of view of the kernel to capture a large context has the disadvantage of increasing the number of computations and parameters to learn. Different from the conventional operation, the atrous convolution operation (Papandreou *et al.*, 2015) can effectively enlarge the field of view of the kernel without suffering the above problems. The newly introduced parameter in atrous convolution is rate r, which controls the spacing in the kernel. It is equivalent to insert $r - 1$ zeros between consecutive elements in the kernel. An example of an atrous convolution operation with $r = 2$ is shown in 6.3(b).

The atrous convolution operation can be formulated as

$$z_{v,u}^{l+1} = \sum_{c=0}^{C^l-1} \sum_{p=0}^{P^l-1} \sum_{q=0}^{Q^l-1} a_{v+r \cdot p, u+r \cdot q, c}^{l} \cdot w_{p,q,c}^{l}. \tag{6.2}$$

It can be seen from 6.2 that atrous convolution is equivalent to standard convolution when $r = 1$. Using atrous convolution in neural network models, it is convenient for us to arbitrarily control the field of view of kernel by setting an appropriate value of r.

6.3.1.2 *Multiple scale features*

Typically, there often exist objects with multiple scales in segmentation tasks. To capture them simultaneously, the traditional method is to resample the input to multiple scales to train the model (Farabet *et al.*, 2012; Lin *et al.*, 2015). However, this approach increases the computational burden significantly. To solve this problem while maintaining the computational cost, ASPP (Chen *et al.*, 2017) is used to extract features with multiple scales from the input directly. ASPP is inspired by spatial pyramid pooling (SPP) (He *et al.*, 2015b), and the main difference between them is the specific operations applied to the input. Specifically, SPP uses multiple pooling operations with different scales to process the input, whereas ASPP uses multiple atrous convolutions. To obtain an intuitive understanding of ASPP, an example of four atrous convolutions with different rates is shown in Fig. 6.4(a). Intuitively, ASPP can be regarded as allowing the model itself to learn the optimal representation of features using multiple atrous convolutions with different rates. The four parallel atrous convolutions are independently applied to the same input to capture features with different scales. After the nonlinear transformation is applied, the output is stacked prior to the next operation. Note that the number of atrous convolutions and their corresponding rates can be customized according to the specific task when applying ASPP in neural network models. The formulation of ASPP is as follows:

$$a^l = \left[a_1^l, \ldots, a_n^l \right]. \tag{6.3}$$

The multiple atrous convolutions in ASPP help capture features with different scales; however, the optimal configuration of ASPP can only

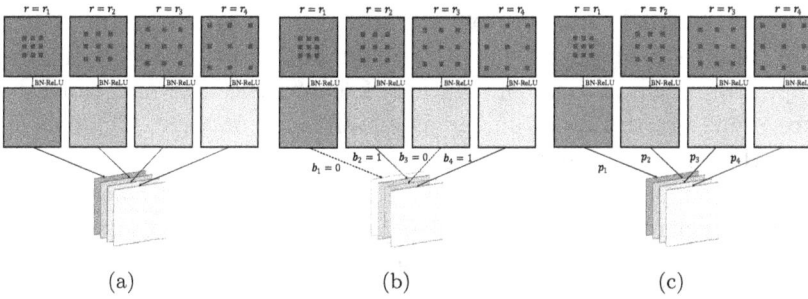

Fig. 6.4. Comparison between ASPP and the proposed sASPP. (a) ASPP is composed of four atrous convolutions with rates ranging from r_1 to r_4. The kernel sizes of all the operations are equal to 3. (b) sASPP in a particular state during the training phase. sASPP has the same rates and kernel size as ASPP shown in (a). The value of b denotes the existence of the feature map, where $b = 0$ denotes the dropped state, and vice versa. (c) sASPP during the test phase. All the feature maps from the atrous convolutions are retained during the test phase, with their magnitude scaled by the retention probability in the training phase.

be determined by trial and error. The question is whether it is possible that the combination of the first m (assuming $m < n$) atrous convolutions perform better than applying all the n operations. Instead of traversing n atrous convolutions to obtain an optimal combination, a novel architecture is proposed that applies randomness to feature maps from atrous convolutions. The motivation and detailed analysis are described in the following section.

6.3.2 *Stochastic atrous spatial pyramid pooling*

6.3.2.1 *Multiple scale features with randomness*

Motivated by stochastic depth networks (Huang *et al.*, 2016), which is a neural network architecture that combines the dropout method (Srivastava *et al.*, 2014) with the residual block in ResNets, a novel method is proposed to regularize ASPP with randomly dropped feature maps from atrous convolutions. Qualitatively, stochastic depth networks can be regarded as a combination of many networks with varying depth because each residual block may be dropped independently, where the proposed architecture can be considered as ASPP with varying width. The proposed architecture is called sASPP because randomness is combined with ASPP. An example of the proposed sASPP during the training phase is shown in 6.4(b). $b_i \in \{0, 1\}$ is a binary variable that controls the existence of feature maps from each atrous convolution. Clearly, the first and third feature maps are dropped, and a^l is equal to $[0, a_2^l, 0, a_4^l]$. Consistent with the dropout technique, scalar variable b_i obeys the Bernoulli distribution parameterized by p_i. This indicates that feature maps from each atrous convolution in ASPP have a probability of p_i of being retained and $1 - p_i$ of being dropped when b_i is one or zero, respectively. Moreover, 6.4 can be reformulated as

$$a^l = \left[b_1 a_1^l, \ldots, b_n a_n^l\right]. \qquad (6.4)$$

Note that the dropout used in sASPP is slightly different from the original dropout method. The dropout here applies independent random variable b_i to the entire feature, rather than to each element of the feature used in the original dropout. This is to consider the complete representation of feature maps from each atrous convolution. p_i is the newly introduced parameter in sASPP and denotes the retained probability of feature maps. The larger the p_i, the greater the contributions by the feature maps from the i-th atrous convolution. The reverse also applies. Intuitively, there are two options for setting p_i. One is to set p_i identically for all the feature maps (e.g., 0.8), which means that they make the same contribution to the segmentation results. The other option is to set p_i as a function of i, which indicates that feature maps from different atrous convolutions contribute unequally according to the size of the field of view. Typically, p_i can increase (or decrease) linearly from p_1 to p_n. The case of linearly increasing p_i is as follows:

$$p_i = p_1 + \frac{p_n - p_1}{n - 1} \cdot (i - 1). \qquad (6.5)$$

The detailed validation of the impact of p_i on the segmentation results is presented in Section 6.4.

6.3.2.2 *Model ensemble*

By applying the stochastic drop operation in ASPP, feature maps from atrous convolutions are likely to be involved in the segmentation. The proposed sASPP can be considered as a combination of 2^n possible networks for the existence status of a_i during the training phase. For the test phase, one possible strategy is to traverse every combination of $\boldsymbol{a}_i$ and average the segmentation output as the final prediction. However, this would significantly increase the computational cost because of the exponential number of models. Following the strategy used in dropout, all the feature maps from atrous convolutions are retained with their values scaled by p_i during the test phase. An example of sASPP during the test phase is shown in 6.4(c). This strategy can be illustrated by combining all possible networks with different widths into a single test architecture, which is an ensemble mechanism. The training and test procedures of sASPP are shown in Algorithm 1. In the training phase, n binary variables are independently sampled from Bernoulli distributions for each mini-batch. $\boldsymbol{a}^{l+1}$ is calculated by concatenating the feature maps multiplied by the binary variables. Note that the stochastic gradient descent algorithm remains the same as that in conventional DNNs. In the test phase, sASPP becomes a deterministic model that uses all the feature maps with their magnitudes scaled by the retention probability.

Algorithm 1: Training and test phases of sASPP.

Require: sASPP with trainable parameters $\boldsymbol{W}$; target $\boldsymbol{y}$; learning rate α

  for training mini-batch j **do**

    for atrous convolution $i \in [1, n]$ **do**

      $\boldsymbol{a}_i^{l+1} \leftarrow F^l(\boldsymbol{W}_i^l * \boldsymbol{a}^l)$

      $b_i \leftarrow Bernoulli\,(p_i)$

    end for

    $\boldsymbol{a}^{l+1} \leftarrow \left[b_1 \boldsymbol{a}_1^{l+1}, \ldots, b_n \boldsymbol{a}_n^{l+1} \right]$

    $\boldsymbol{W} \leftarrow \boldsymbol{W} - \alpha \frac{\partial C(\boldsymbol{a}^L, \boldsymbol{y})}{\partial \boldsymbol{W}}$

  end for

  for test sample j **do**

    for atrous convolution $i \in [1, n]$ **do**

      $\boldsymbol{a}_i^{l+1} \leftarrow F^l(\boldsymbol{W}_i^l * \boldsymbol{a}^l)$

    end for

    $\boldsymbol{a}^{l+1} \leftarrow \left[p_1 \boldsymbol{a}_1^{l+1}, \ldots, p_n \boldsymbol{a}_n^{l+1} \right]$

  end for

6.4   Experimental Setup and Results

In this section, the experimental setup is presented, including the dataset and specific configuration of the proposed method. Then, the results of control experiments are given and analyzed in detail.

6.4.1   *Experimental setup*

6.4.1.1   *Dataset*

The dataset is sourced from a competition platform called AI Challenger which is hosted by several well-known Internet enterprises in China. The dataset is well annotated at the pixel level. SRF and PED lesions are used to validate our proposed method. The dataset is composed of training, validation, and test parts that contain 70, 15, and 15 cases, respectively. Each case contains 128 slices, with a resolution of 512×1024. Note that only the training and validation datasets' annotations have been released. The team that participated in the challenge is required to train and assess its model using the training and validation dataset, and upload the segmentation prediction on the test dataset. The final rank on the leaderboard is based on the comparison between the uploaded prediction with the ground truth of the test dataset. There are two rounds in the challenge, namely round A and B. We won the first and second places in the two rounds, respectively. The test datasets in both rounds are the same, and the difference relies on the updates of the leaderboard. In round A, the participants can upload their prediction results three times per week and the score is updated immediately. In round B, there are totally two chances to upload the prediction results, while the score is invisible until the end of the challenge. The final score in each round is based on the highest one. The leaderboard is shown in Table 6.1. Because the annotations of the test dataset in the competition are not provided, the models in the following experiments are evaluated on the validation dataset.

6.4.1.2   *Configurations*

ASPP and the proposed sASPP are types of modules that aim to extract features with multiple fields of view. To evaluate

Table 6.1.   The leaderboard of macular edema segmentation competition in AI Challenger. The score is calculated by the mean DSC value of each lesion type.

Team	Score of Round A	Team	Score of Round B
Our	**0.7521**	965728310	0.7612
965728310	0.7466	**Our**	**0.7521**
Looking	0.7458	Looking	0.7460
DeepSeg	0.7441	Viking	0.7442
Menelvagor	0.7398	DeepSeg	0.7441

their performance on the macular edema segmentation task, the DeepLabv3+ (Chen *et al.*, 2018) model combined with ASPP or sASPP is used. DeepLab is a series of segmentation models that have achieved state-of-the-art performance on the PASCAL VOC 2012 semantic segmentation task. DeepLabv3+ is the most recent model that has delivered better performance than the previous series models. The distinction between DeepLabv3+ and the other versions is the encoder and decoder paradigm. Specifically, a backbone network (e.g., ResNet or Xception) together with atrous convolutions is used as the encoder. The decoder part uses the low-level features from the middle part of the encoder and outputs of ASPP to obtain the final segmentation results. In this study, a 1×1 convolution together with three atrous convolutions with the kernel size of 3×3 (rates are 6, 12, and 18) are used in ASPP and sASPP. ResNet50 is used as the backbone network. sASPP with three configurations are used in the control experiments, including linearly increased, decreased, and identical values of p_i, which are denoted as sASPP $(p \uparrow)$, sASPP $(p \downarrow)$, and sASPP $(p = 0.8)$, respectively. p_i in the three configurations are $\{0.5, 0.6, 0.7, 0.8\}$, $\{0.8, 0.7, 0.6, 0.5\}$, and $\{0.8, 0.8, 0.8, 0.8\}$. For ReLayNet, the implementation is based on the open-source code provided by the original authors.[1] For 3D U-Net, we implement the network structure that is described in (De Fauw *et al.*, 2018).

---

[1]https://github.com/ai-med/relaynet_pytorch.

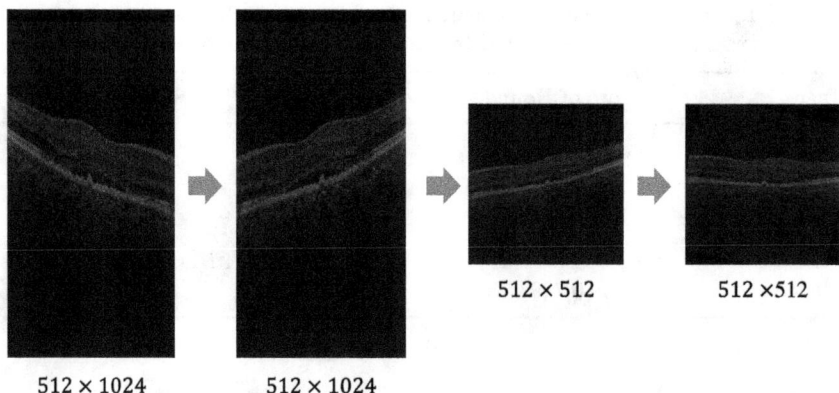

Fig. 6.5.   Data augmentation pipeline in the training phase. The number below each image denotes the width and height. From left to right are the original, horizontal flipped, resized, and rotated images. All the operations are randomly performed.

The size of the raw input is 512×1024, which is too large for the model. To alleviate the computational burden, the size of the input is set to 512×512 during the training phase. The dataset in the training phase is extensively augmented to mitigate the problem of overfitting. The augmentation pipeline is shown in Fig. 6.5. Note that the resize augmentation represented by the third image is composed of random scale and crop/padding operations. If the output of the scale operation is larger than 512, then the image is cropped to 512; otherwise it is padded with zeros. In the experiments, the scale ratio is in $[0.75, 1.5]$ and the maximum rotation angle is 15. At the end of the augmentation pipeline, the data are divided by 255 to ensure the pixel values are located in $[0, 1]$.

DeepLabv3+ with ASPP or sASPP is trained with the backpropagation algorithm by minimizing the cross-entropy cost function with respect to the parameters

$$\mathcal{J} = -\frac{1}{M} \sum_{m=1}^{M} \boldsymbol{y}_m^{\top} \ln(\boldsymbol{a}_m^L), \qquad (6.6)$$

where M denotes the number of images in a batch and $\boldsymbol{a}^L$ denotes the output of the model after applying the softmax function. To optimize the above cost function, stochastic gradient descent with momentum algorithm is used. The learning rate and momentum are set to 1×10^{-7} and 0.9, respectively. L2 regularization with the weight decay 5×10^{-4} is also used. The number of images in each batch is 10, and the training process is completed when 60 epochs is reached.

The true positive volume fraction (TPVF), positive predictive value (PPV), and dice similarity coefficient (DSC) are used to evaluate the model's performance. These metrics have been widely used to assess the performance of segmentation tasks (Udupa *et al.*, 2006; Papandreou *et al.*, 2015; Roy *et al.*, 2017; Xu *et al.*, 2017). Their definitions are as follows:

$$\text{TPVF} = \frac{|V_S \cap V_G|}{|V_G|}, \tag{6.7}$$

$$\text{PPV} = \frac{|V_S \cap V_G|}{|V_S|}, \tag{6.8}$$

$$\text{DSC} = 2 \times \frac{|V_S \cap V_G|}{|V_S \cup V_G|}, \tag{6.9}$$

where V_S and V_G denote the volume of the model's segmentation results and ground truth, respectively.

6.4.1.3 *Implementation*

The proposed model is implemented using PyTorch (Paszke *et al.*, 2017). All experiments are carried out on a server with Linux OS and hardware of CPU Intel Xeon E5-2620 @2.4GHz, four NVIDIA Tesla K40m GPUs, and 64 GB of RAM.

6.4.2 *Results*

6.4.2.1 *Comparison with the state of the art*

The quantitative comparison between ASPP, ReLayNet, and 3D U-Net is described as follows. Table 6.2 shows the values of the three metrics for the segmentation of SRF and PED lesions. For the segmentation of SRF, the ASPP demonstrates significantly superior performance compared with ReLayNet and 3D U-Net. The DSC of

Table 6.2. Performance comparison between ReLayNet, 3D U-Net, and ASPP in the segmentation of SRF and PED lesions.

| Model | SRF | | |
	DSC	TPVF	PPV
ReLayNet	0.5472 ± 0.10	0.4550 ± 0.10	0.6862 ± 0.09
3D U-Net	0.8060 ± 0.08	0.7328 ± 0.12	$\mathbf{0.8954} \pm 0.07$
ASPP	$\mathbf{0.8447} \pm 0.07$	$\mathbf{0.8214} \pm 0.11$	0.8693 ± 0.09

| Model | PED | | |
	DSC	TPVF	PPV
ReLayNet	0.5820 ± 0.13	0.6224 ± 0.16	$\mathbf{0.5464} \pm 0.14$
3D U-Net	0.6131 ± 0.11	0.7785 ± 0.17	0.5057 ± 0.07
ASPP	$\mathbf{0.6370} \pm 0.09$	$\mathbf{0.8341} \pm 0.10$	0.5153 ± 0.11

Note: The bold numbers indicate the best results for each performance index.

ASPP is 0.8447, which is over 0.5472 and 0.8060 in ReLayNet and 3D U-Net by a large margin. The advantages of ASPP can be also observed in the metrics of TPVF, where ASPP achieves higher scores than ReLayNet and 3D U-Net. The 3D U-Net achieves the highest PPV score which is 0.8954 among the three models. For the segmentation of PED, the DSC score of ASPP is 0.6370, which is still higher than 0.5820 and 0.6131 in ReLayNet and 3D U-Net, respectively. For the TPVF metric, ASPP substantially exceeds ReLayNet and 3D U-Net where the values for ASPP, ReLayNet, and 3D U-Net are 0.8341, 0.6224, and 0.7785, respectively. The higher score demonstrates that ASPP can recognize more PED lesions compared with the other two models. However, the PPV in ASPP is 0.5153, which is inferior to 0.5464 in ReLayNet. The lower PPV score in ASPP indicates that the positive samples predicted by ASPP are more prone to be incorrect than those in ReLayNet. In terms of ASPP, the low PPV score also causes the DSC score in the segmentation of PED to be much lower than that in SRF because the DSC is a balanced metric that is determined by TPVF and PPV simultaneously. These quantitative experimental results indicate that ASPP performs much better than ReLayNet and 3D U-Net on the SRF and PED segmentation tasks. To further validate the effectiveness of ASPP, we also carry out experiment on the fluid segmentation task of Duke dataset (Chiu *et al.*, 2015) for which ReLayNet reported their results. The split of training and test datasets is kept the same as the one in (Roy *et al.*, 2017). The DSC, TPVF, and PPV scores of ASPP are 0.8025 ± 0.04, 0.8619 ± 0.08, and 0.7490 ± 0.02, respectively. The DSC score of ASPP is higher than the reported 0.77 of ReLayNet.

In the following, we qualitatively compare the segmentation results of ASPP, 3D U-Net, and ReLayNet. The ground truth together with the prediction of ASPP, 3D U-Net, and ReLayNet of five OCT slices are shown in Fig. 6.6. It can be seen that all the three methods accurately segment the SRF lesions in the first slice. For the second slice, ASPP identifies the majority of the SRF lesions, except the precise segmentation of the anomalous boundaries, which is mainly caused by the built-in transformation invariance ability in deep convolutional neural networks. Both the 3D U-Net and ReLayNet only identify a small part of the lesion. The same result can be observed in the third slice. In the fourth slice, the segmentation results of ASPP and 3D U-Net are closer to the ground truth than those of ReLayNet. Moreover, ReLayNet misclassifies a small portion of PED to SRF. Both the three methods recognize the majority of the SRF lesions in the fifth slice. However, ReLayNet fails to recognize the PED lesions.

The superiority of ASPP can be attributed to the following two reasons: First, a key factor in the segmentation task are the effective features that can fully represent lesions. Note that the input of ASPP are the highly abstract features produced from ResNet50. Compared with ResNet50, the encoder network in both ReLayNet and 3D U-Net has a much shallow depth. Second, the multiple atrous convolutions in ASPP can capture the features in multiple scales, which is favorable in macular edema segmentation tasks. However, the relatively shallow depth of the encoder network and the fixed size of convolution kernel in ReLayNet and 3D U-Net may impede the model's ability to extract features from lesions of various shapes and sizes.

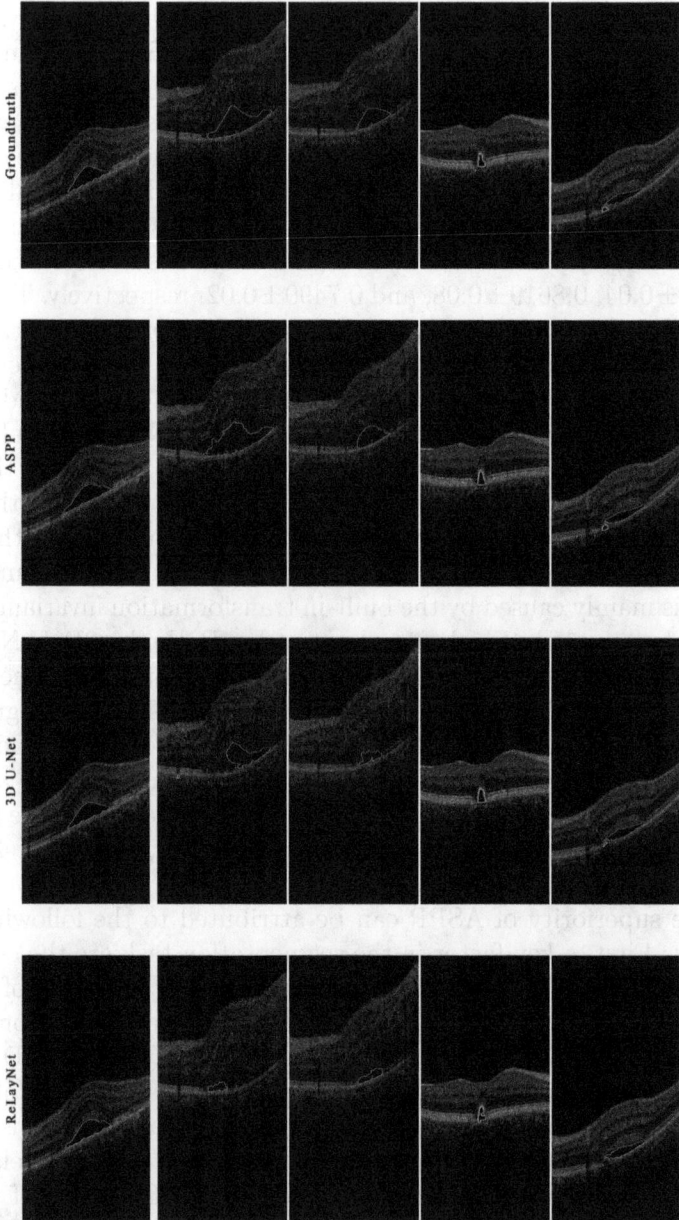

Fig. 6.6. Qualitative comparison between ASPP, 3D U-Net, and ReLayNet. The four rows denote the ground truth, prediction results of ASPP, 3D U-Net, and ReLayNet. Each column represents a specific slice in OCT.

6.4.2.2   *Stochastic atrous spatial pyramid pooling*

The performance comparison between ASPP and sASPP is described as follows. Table 6.3 shows the quantitative segmentation results of ASPP and sASPP. As can be seen in the Table 6.3, sASPP ($p \uparrow$) achieves higher scores than ASPP in the segmentation of SRF. sASPP ($p \uparrow$) also obtains a higher DSC score in the segmentation of PED. However, this superiority mainly benefits from the higher PPV score, where the values in sASPP ($p \uparrow$) and ASPP are 0.6975 and 0.5153, respectively. In terms of the TPVF, the value in sASPP ($p \uparrow$) is 0.6705, which is much lower than 0.8341 in ASPP. The performance of sASPP ($p \downarrow$) is also evaluated, which is shown in the third line of Table 6.3. Contrary to sASPP ($\uparrow$), sASPP ($\downarrow$) achieves a lower DSC score compared with ASPP in the segmentation of SRF. For the segmentation of PED, sASPP ($p \downarrow$) achieves a higher DSC score compared with both ASPP and sASPP ($p \uparrow$).

Note that sASPP randomly drops the feature maps produced from the atrous convolutions during training phase, where parameter p denotes the retained probability. A larger value of p indicates that the corresponding atrous convolution plays a more important role. For sASPP ($p \uparrow$) and sASPP ($p \downarrow$), the atrous convolution with large and small fields of view dominates the segmentation results. Based on the DSC scores of ASPP and sASPP with linear variation, it can be observed that the large and small fields of view matter in the segmentation of SRF and PED lesions, respectively. To further verify the effectiveness of parameter p, all the retained probabilities of the feature maps are set to 0.8 and the results are shown in the last row

Table 6.3.   Performance comparison between ASPP and sASPP with different configurations.

Model	SRF			PED		
	DSC	TPVF	PPV	DSC	TPVF	PPV
ASPP	0.8447	0.8214	0.8693	0.637	**0.8341**	0.5153
sASPP ($p \uparrow$)	0.8716	0.8648	0.8785	0.6837	0.6705	**0.6975**
sASPP ($p \downarrow$)	0.8166	0.7557	**0.8881**	0.7189	0.8255	0.6368
sASPP ($p = 0.8$)	**0.8759**	**0.8799**	0.8719	**0.7371**	0.8147	0.6729

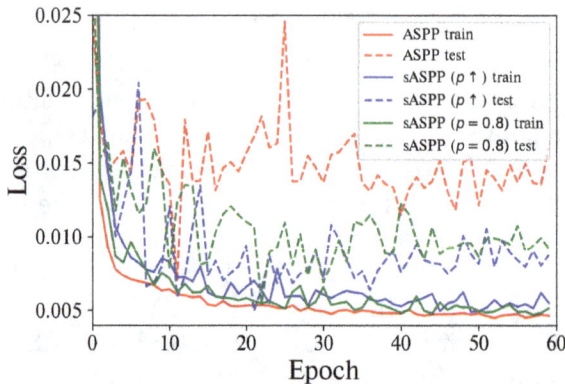

Fig. 6.7.   Comparison of training and test losses between ASPP and sASPP.

of Table 6.3. We find that sASPP ($p = 0.8$) achieves the highest DSC score among all the models in both segmentations of SRF and PED.

A qualitative comparison of the convergence speed between ASPP and sASPP is also performed. The training and test losses in each epoch are shown in Fig. 6.7. It can be seen that the training loss of ASPP decreases the fastest among the three models, whereas sASPP ($p \uparrow$) decreases slightly faster than sASPP ($p = 0.8$). Note that the training loss in sASPP oscillates much more than that in ASPP, which is partially caused by sASPP's adaption to the various possible combinations of feature maps in the training phase. Moreover, contrary convergence results in terms of test loss can be observed. The order of methods with respect to the test errors, from low to high, is sASPP ($p \uparrow$), sASPP ($p = 0.8$), and ASPP. Compared with ASPP, sASPP achieves lower test errors whereas the training errors also decrease slower. In terms of the gap between training and test losses, it is clear to observe that the one in sASPP is much smaller than that in ASPP. These convergence results demonstrate that the stochastic drop operation is an effective regularization method that can alleviate the overfitting problem in the segmentation task.

The Bland–Altman plots which measure the limits of agreement of SRF and PED are shown in Fig. 6.8. The voxel size of the OCT data is $12 \times 47 \times 1.95$ um^3. It is noted that the volume of SRF is much larger than that of PED in the dataset. It can be seen that the

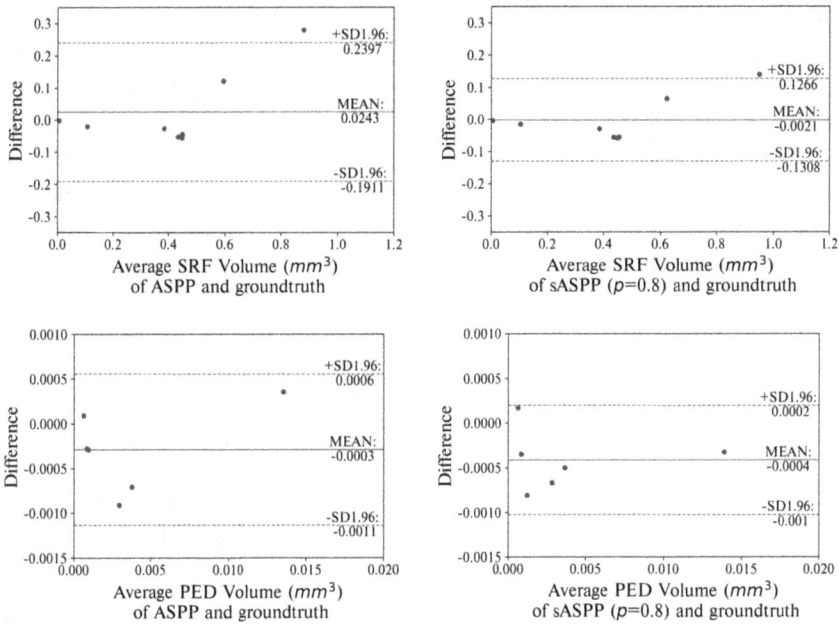

Fig. 6.8. The Bland–Altman plots which measure the limits of agreement of SRF and PED.

95% limits of agreement between sASPP and ground truth are narrower than those between ASPP and ground truth in both SRF and PED. Moreover, the average discrepancy between sASPP and ground truth in the lesion of SRF is -0.0027, which is smaller than 0.0307 between ASPP and ground truth in terms of the absolute value. For the lesion of PED, the absolute average discrepancy between sASPP and ground truth is larger than that between ASPP and ground truth. It might be caused by the lower TPVF value of sASPP when compared with ASPP.

6.4.2.3 *Analytical experiment*

To empirically validate the importance of atrous convolutions in ASPP and sASPP, control experiments are carried out using gradually enabled atrous convolutions. The DSC scores are shown in

Table 6.4. For ASPP, the DSC score of the SRF monotonically increases when more atrous convolutions are involved. This uptrend for SRF can be also observed in the model of sASPP with different settings of p, which indicates all the four components in ASPP contribute to the segmentation of SRF. However, these contributions are unequally distributed. It can be seen that the increment of the DSC score caused by the introduction of $r = 18$ is less than that for $r = 6$. For sASPP ($p \uparrow$) and sASPP ($p = 0.8$), the DSC score is very low when only using atrous convolutions with $r = 1$ or $r = 6$, which is mainly caused by the intensity scale mechanism during the test phase.

For ASPP in the segmentation of PED, the model achieves the highest DSC score when atrous convolutions with $r = 1$ and $r = 6$ are involved. Introducing atrous convolution with a large rate (e.g., $r = 12$ or $r = 16$) in ASPP decreases the DSC score. This negative impact is alleviated in sASPP, where all DSC scores

Table 6.4. DSC score of ASPP and sASPP with different combinations of atrous convolutions. A tick denotes the involvement of atrous convolution.

Model	$r = 1$	$r = 6$	$r = 12$	$r = 18$	DSC SRF	DSC PED
ASPP	✓				0.5812	0.5745
ASPP	✓	✓			0.7862	0.6674
ASPP	✓	✓	✓		0.8312	0.6525
ASPP	✓	✓	✓	✓	0.8447	0.6370
sASPP ($p \uparrow$)	✓				0.0051	0.0134
sASPP ($p \uparrow$)	✓	✓			0.6192	0.0364
sASPP ($p \uparrow$)	✓	✓	✓		0.8351	0.4287
sASPP ($p \uparrow$)	✓	✓	✓	✓	0.8716	0.6837
sASPP ($p \downarrow$)	✓				0.6886	0.3482
sASPP ($p \downarrow$)	✓	✓			0.7867	0.7032
sASPP ($p \downarrow$)	✓	✓	✓		0.7978	0.7303
sASPP ($p \downarrow$)	✓	✓	✓	✓	0.8166	0.7189
sASPP ($p = 0.8$)	✓				0.4164	0.0115
sASPP ($p = 0.8$)	✓	✓			0.8131	0.5120
sASPP ($p = 0.8$)	✓	✓	✓		0.8639	0.7189
sASPP ($p = 0.8$)	✓	✓	✓	✓	0.8759	0.7371

Table 6.5.   Performance comparison between ASPP and sASPP on 3DIRCADb.

Model	Liver			Tumor		
	DSC	TPVF	PPV	DSC	TPVF	PPV
ASPP	0.9432 ± 0.01	0.9591 ± 0.02	$\mathbf{0.9278} \pm 0.01$	0.6258 ± 0.01	0.4911 ± 0.13	$\mathbf{0.8624} \pm 0.11$
sASPP ($p = 0.8$)	$\mathbf{0.9486} \pm 0.01$	$\mathbf{0.9706} \pm 0.02$	0.9275 ± 0.02	$\mathbf{0.6774} \pm 0.008$	$\mathbf{0.5714} \pm 0.09$	0.8314 ± 0.11

in the segmentation of PED monotonically increase, except for $r = 18$ in sASPP ($p \downarrow$). The above results demonstrate that sASPP can use the atrous convolutions with multiple rates better than ASPP.

6.4.2.4 *Comparison on 3DIRCADb dataset*

To further validate the generalization of the proposed method, 3DIRCADb dataset (Soler *et al.*, 2010), which contains 3D CT scans of livers and lesions, is further used to conduct experiments. The dataset includes 20 volumes where 15 of them contain hepatic tumors. Among those 15 volumes, 5 and 10 volumes are used as test and training datasets, respectively. Two tasks are performed, including the segmentation of livers and tumors. Table 6.5 shows the segmentation performance of ASPP and sASPP ($p = 0.8$). For the segmentation of the liver, it can be seen that the sASPP achieves higher DSC and TPVF scores compared with ASPP. The superiority of sASPP can be also observed in the segmentation of tumors in terms of the DSC and TPVF scores. However, the PPV score of ASPP in the segmentation of tumor is higher than that of sASPP. Furthermore, Fig. 6.9 shows the qualitative comparison of segmentation results between sASPP and ASPP. For the first two scans, it can be seen that both the ASPP and sASPP have accurately segment the livers and tumors. For the third scan, the ASPP wrongly segments a small part of normal tissues into tumors, where the sASPP segments correctly. These results further demonstrate the effectiveness and robustness of the proposed method.

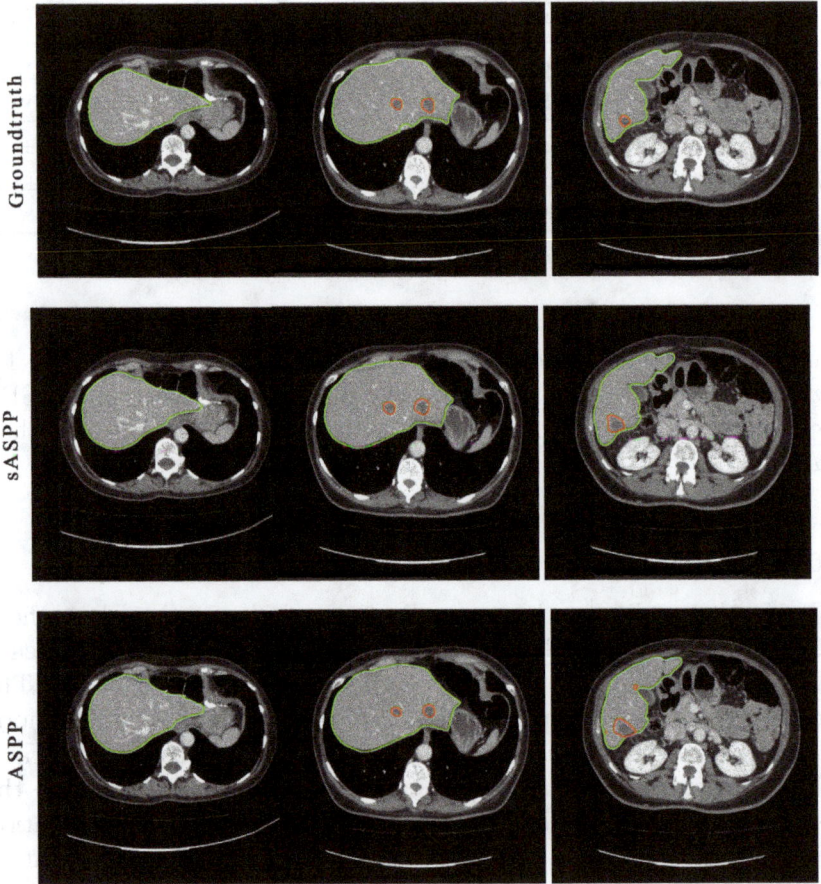

Fig. 6.9. Qualitative comparison between sASPP and ASPP. The three rows denote the ground truth and prediction results of sASPP and ASPP. Each column represents a specific scan in a CT volume. The red and green lines represent the edges of livers and tumors.

6.5 DeepOCT: An AI System for Macular Edema Lesion Segmentation

Thanks to the advantages of fast speed, non-invasive, and high accuracy, OCT has become one of the most important examination methods for macular edema in clinic. It can accurately display the stratification information of the patient's fundus retina. Ophthalmologists can quantitatively evaluate the condition of the patient's fundus by observing the OCT image, so as to give a more objective diagnosis conclusion. However, since a single OCT examination will generate tens to hundreds of tomographic images, it will be a time-consuming and laborious work for doctors to manually examine and judge the macular edema area one by one.

Based on this, we have developed an intelligent auxiliary diagnosis system called DeepOCT for macular edema lesions, which is oriented to ophthalmologists. The system aims to automatically segment the macular edema lesions from the OCT images of patients according to the established deep neural network segmentation model, so as to assist ophthalmologists in quantitatively diagnosing the lesions.

The DeepOCT is a B/S architecture. The server is deployed on the Alibaba Cloud public network and is mainly responsible for data management and model calculation. The overall architecture of the system is shown in Fig. 6.10. The doctor only needs to upload multiple OCT images examined by the patient to the cloud server using the browser. After receiving the data, the server will complete the lesion segmentation one by one using the trained deep neural network segmentation model and return the segmentation results to the client browser. After receiving the segmentation result, the client will identify different macular edema focus areas by color and support editing the segmentation result.

After logging into the system, click the "select file" button in Fig. 6.11 to select the OCT cases to be divided from the local folder.

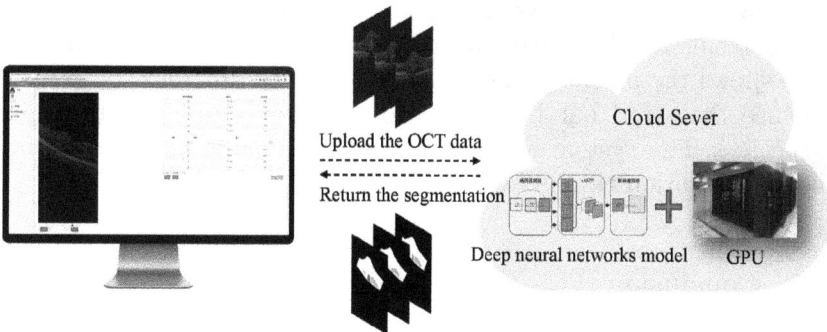

Fig. 6.10.   The system architecture of DeepOCT.

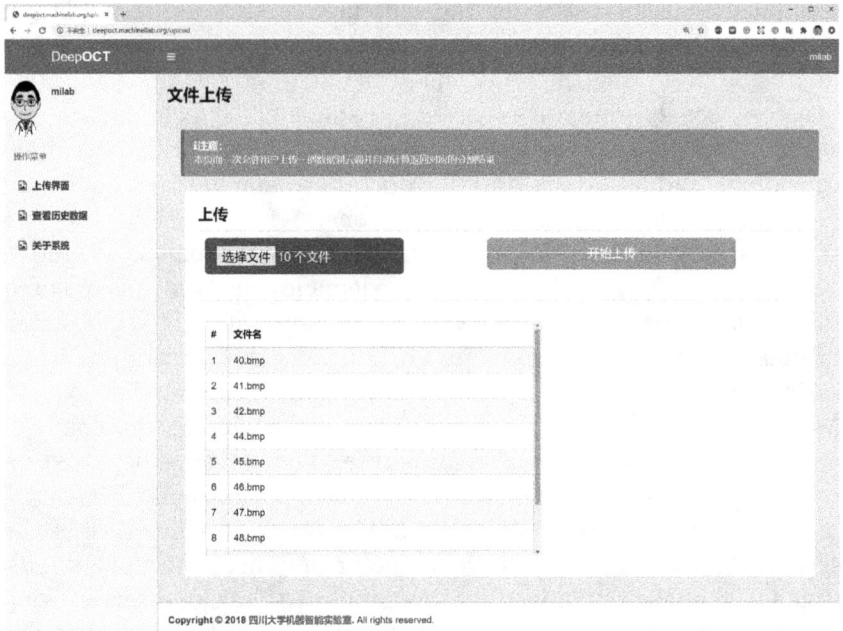

Fig. 6.11.   Data upload page in DeepOCT.

After selection, the OCT slices to be uploaded included in the case will be listed at the bottom of the page. Click "start uploading"; the client will automatically upload the case to the cloud server and display the data uploading progress in real time. After receiving the uploaded OCT image, the server will use the trained macular edema lesion segmentation model to predict the lesion area slice by slice. After all slices are predicted, the browser will jump to the segmentation result display page shown in Fig. 6.12. The left side of the page shows the macular edema focus area with different colors. You can use the scroll bar below to slide to view the segmentation of each slice. The system also supports editing, adding, and deleting the segmentation results of the focus.

6.6   Conclusion

In this chapter, an encoder–decoder model together with ASPP is used to segment SRF and PED lesions in OCT images. The encoder

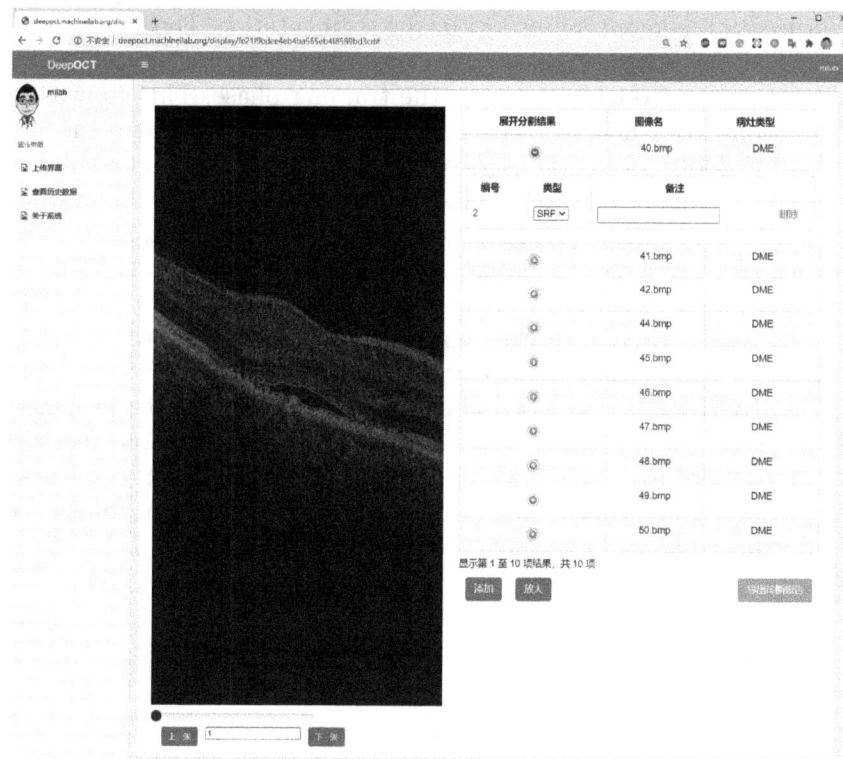

Fig. 6.12.   The segmentation results in DeepOCT.

is based on ResNet50, which has a large capacity to learn to extract high-level features of lesions from the raw OCT image. Then, the features are fed into ASPP, which is composed of multiple atrous convolutions with different rates. Benefiting from the advantages of atrous convolution, ASPP effectively processes the features by applying various fields of view without increasing the computational cost and learnable parameters. The experimental results demonstrate that ASPP is favorable in the macular edema segmentation task and substantially outperformed the state-of-the-art model.

A novel module called sASPP, which combines randomness with ASPP, is further proposed. sASPP stochastically drops the feature maps produced by the atrous convolutions in ASPP during the training phase. The retained probability of each feature map is equivalent to its contribution, where the larger probability represents the feature map is more important in the segmentation. During the test phase, all the feature maps are retained, with their intensity scaled by the retention probability during the training phase. This stochastic operation is an effective ensemble mechanism to prevent the co-adaptation of multiple atrous convolutions in ASPP. The results of the control experiments indicate that the various atrous convolutions are non-equivalent in the segmentation of SRF and PED. The atrous convolutions with large fields of view are more preferable in the segmentation of SRF than that of PED. Compared with ASPP, the proposed sASPP further improves the DSC score while maintaining a significantly lower error on the test dataset. Experiments on 3DIRCADb dataset also validate the superiority of the proposed sASPP. In future studies, we intent to apply the proposed method to more types of macular edema related lesions. Additionally, learning mechanisms will be integrated into sASPP to better adjust the importance of the multiple atrous convolutions.

Chapter 7

DeepUWF: An Automated Ultrawide-field Fundus Screening System via Deep Learning

The emerging ultrawide field of view (UWF) fundus color imaging is a powerful tool for fundus screening. However, manual screening is labor-intensive and subjective. Based on 2644 UWF images, a set of early fundus abnormal screening systems named DeepUWF is developed. DeepUWF includes an abnormal fundus screening subsystem and a disease diagnosis subsystem for three kinds of fundus diseases (retinal tear and retinal detachment, diabetic retinopathy, and pathological myopia). The components in the system are composed of a set of excellent convolutional neural networks and two custom classifiers. However, the contrast of UWF images used in the research is low, which seriously limits the extraction of fine features of UWF images by depth model. Therefore, the high specificity and low sensitivity of prediction results have always been difficult problems in research. In order to solve this problem, six kinds of image preprocessing techniques are adopted, and their effects on the prediction performance of fundus abnormal and three kinds of fundus disease models are studied. A variety of experimental indicators are used to evaluate the algorithms for validity and reliability. The experimental results show that these preprocessing methods are helpful to improve the learning ability of the networks and achieve good sensitivity and specificity. Without ophthalmologists, DeepUWF has potential application value, which is helpful for fundus health screening and workflow improvement.

7.1 Introduction

Visual impairment is one of the major health problems in the world (World Health Organization *et al.*, 2019, 2013). At present, more than 2.2 billion people are blind or visually impaired in the world, including nearly 55 million in China. Besides, by 2050, the aging and growing global population could triple the number of blind people. The main reasons for visual impairment are lifestyle factors and limited eye care resources (Rra *et al.*, 2017; Bourne *et al.*, 2013; Li-xin, 2017; Chi, 2012). Therefore, early screening and timely treatment are the keys to prevent vision damage. However, even if telemedicine can be provided in low-income and middle-income areas, the increase in misdiagnosis and missed diagnosis rate of telemedicine mean that time-consuming and laborious manual screening cannot be ignored (Singh *et al.*, 2014; Berwick *et al.*, 2012; Zhao *et al.*, 2010).

Ophthalmology is a field which is highly dependent on fundus imaging technology. Compared with traditional fundus color imaging providing $30°-75°$ views, the new ultrawide-field imaging technology (UWF) can provide the largest retina area with $200°$ views, which is very important in the detection of peripheral retinal lesions by locating lesions based on imaging (Fig. 7.1(a)) (Wessel *et al.*, 2012; Soliman *et al.*, 2012; Silva *et al.*, 2016).

There is a broad consensus in western countries that UWF imaging technology can bring great public health benefits because it may make hospitals only serve those patients who really need tertiary care (Nagiel *et al.*, 2016; Falavarjani *et al.*, 2016; Fenner *et al.*, 2018). However, in China, limited retinal experts and well-trained readers are the main problems of applying these better retinal views.

Encouragingly, deep learning (DL), especially convolutional neural networks (CNNs), has shown outstanding performance in recent medical research (Esteva *et al.*, 2017; Chen and Davies, 2020; Qi *et al.*, 2019), especially in the field of ophthalmology (Gulshan *et al.*, 2016; He *et al.*, 2019). CNNs can directly extract knowledge from labeled original images without human intervention (Bengio *et al.*, 2013; LeCun *et al.*, 2015; Yi, 2010). Three driving forces to promote

DL medical integration are as follows: (1) using remote diagnosis and treatment systems to expand the coverage of screening projects and reduce the entry barriers in areas with scarce medical resources; (2) improving the efficiency and repeatability of diagnosis; (3) improving the accuracy of referral and reducing the overall medical costs by early interventions of treatable diseases, so as to prevent expensive interventions afterwards (Abràmoff *et al.*, 2018; Greenspan *et al.*, 2016).

Therefore, in this study, an automatic system called DeepUWF is developed, which aims to provide clinical reference when retinal experts are scarce. The system includes two steps: screening UWF photos to determine the existence of abnormal fundus and reporting clinical tests. The contributions of this work are as follows:

(1) A database containing 2644 UWF images is established.
(2) Six UWF image optimization methods are used to study the classification performance of fundus anomalies and three fundus disease models.
(3) An UWF fundus screening system is developed, which is used to identify the presence or absence of abnormal fundus and diagnose three fundus diseases, including retinal tear and retinal detachment (RT&RD), diabetic retinopathy (DR), and myopia.

The outline of this paper is as follows: In Section 7.2, we analyze the relevant works. In Section 7.3, we describe the dataset in detail. In Section 7.4, we discuss the system. In Section 7.5, we introduce the experiment in detail. In Section 7.6, we provide a discussion of the whole research and future work. Finally, in Section 7.7, we come to the conclusion.

7.2 Related Works

7.2.1 *Deep learning with traditional imaging technology*

Ophthalmology research related to DL has developed vigorously recently. Color fundus imaging, as one traditional fundus imaging mode, has commonly been used in DL diagnosis of retinal diseases recently. Some DL architectures for determining the color mode have been trained from scratch (Pratt *et al.*, 2016; Abràmoff *et al.*, 2016), whereas better predictive performance has been achieved by networks trained via transfer learning (Kaggle, 2016; Ting *et al.*, 2017; Zhang *et al.*, 2019). Li *et al.* proposed a DL model for detecting referable glaucomatous optic neuropathy. It is trained on 48,116 images and has high sensitivity (95.6%) and specificity (92.0%) (Li *et al.*, 2018). More remarkably, the first AI-based auxiliary DR screening system, IDX-DR, is authorized by the FDA for marketing in April 2018 (Topol, 2019).

One potential difficulty with the aforementioned projects is that this imaging method cannot be fully recognized and judged by the automatic detection system because of its inability to observe the peripheral region.

7.2.2 *Deep learning with emerging UWF imaging technology*

UWF imaging has broken this bottleneck because of its wide imaging range, and it is a powerful tool for outpatient fundus screening, having gradually changed the classification and management of certain fundus diseases. Ohsuqi *et al.* showed that DL technology is better for the detection of branch retinal vein occlusions using 466 images (Nagasato *et al.*, 2019). Matsuba *et al.* proposed a DL system to detect AMD, with a high sensitivity and specificity of 100% and 97.31% respectively based on 364 UWF images (Matsuba *et al.*, 2019). Hiroki *et al.* developed a DL model to detect and grade glaucoma on 1399 UWF images, and it had AUCs of 87.2% and 93.4% (Hiroki *et al.*, 2018). Those studies mainly focused on the diagnosis of certain fundus ophthalmopathy.

7.3 Dataset

7.3.1 *Materials*

The UWF data are retrospectively collected between June 2018 and November 2019 at three hospitals in China. Among that, 1512 UWF retinal images are obtained from a high-ranking physical examination (PE) center in Sichuan Province, 446 UWF images are contained from the Ophthalmology Department of Sichuan Provincial People's Hospital (SP), and 686 UWF images are obtained from Zhongshan

Ophthalmology Department (ZS). The two latter hospitals often receive patients with various refractory retinal diseases from different places, thus images from the hospitals are more challenging.

7.3.2 Annotation standard

To facilitate the high-quality labeling of images, a special UWF data labeling system is developed and includes the following steps: first, the annotator evaluates the image quality. If it is difficult or impossible for the annotators to reliably judge the presence of pathological features, the image is deleted. Second, the annotator estimates each image based on the two aspects of abnormal sign description or proposed fundus disease opinion. Third, the annotator can mark the images as normal or abnormal according to the above conclusion. Table 7.1 shows details of the assessment.

The annotators include a retinal specialist with more than 30 years of research experience and three certified ophthalmologists, each with at least five years of clinical experience. The final label result must be agreed upon among the three retinal specialists, and any objection is arbitrated by the senior retinal specialist.

7.3.3 Annotation result

The labeling results show that the abnormal signs of images are diverse; moreover, the fundus diseases mainly fall into the following four categories: RT, RD, DR, and myopia, which are the main causes of visual impairment or blindness worldwide. Besides, considering that the number of RT is limited and it can cause RD, we currently classify the two diseases as the same screening target. In general, data from PE showed that nearly 87% of the examinees had no obvious signs of abnormality in the fundus. Nearly four-fifths of ZS patients are diagnosed with fundus abnormalities, and RT&RD is the main fundus disease. Half of the examiners from SP are diagnosed with fundus abnormalities, and the possibility of myopia in the diagnosis of further fundus diseases is about 79.5%. Moreover, some images contain multi-disease labels, but they are not included in the study of major diseases due to the wide distribution of diseases and limited sample size (e.g., cataract, glaucoma, AMD, AH, and MF). Finally, we obtain a total of 2,644 labeled images used

Table 7.1. Details of annotation standard.

Sign area	Possible lesions or disease categories
OND	Optic disc atrophy, Blurred optic disc boundary, Optic disc dysplasia, Cup disc ratio increases, Pigmented patches atrophic rings, and Others.
Retinopathy	Retinal artery tortuosity, Retinal vein tortuosity, Retinal vascular occlusion or white sheath, Retinal hemorrhage, Retinal exudation, RT, RD, Peripheral retinal degeneration area, Peripheral retinal, Retinal pigmentation (or proliferation), Proliferating membrane, Neovascularization, Regional abnormal color, Loss of retinal pigment, Retinitis pigmentosa, Yellow-white lesions, and Others.
Maculopathy	Macular hemorrhage, Macular exudation, Macular hole, Epimacular membrane, Macular choroidal atrophy, Yellow-white lesions, and Others.
VPC	Vitreous hemorrhage, Asteroid hyalosis (AH), Vitreous opacity, Vitreous floaters, and Others.
Other	Refractive media turbidity, Myelinated nerve fiber, Postoperation, and Others.
Disease	DR, Myopia, Cataract, AMD, Glaucoma, RD, RT, Macular edema, Papilledema, Vitreous hemorrhage, Space occupying lesion, Medullated fibers (MF), Choroid atrophy in macular area, Optic papilla atrophy, Central retinal vein occlusion (or artery), and Others.

Notes: OND: optic nerve damages, VPC: vitreous pathologic change.

for the screening system and 899 labeled images used for the disease diagnosis system. Table 7.2 provides detailed statistics regarding the distribution of images among categories.

7.3.4 *Preprocessing of UWF images*

According to the guidelines of "Operation and Reading Specifications of Ultrawide-field Fundus Imaging Technology in China (2018)", when evaluating imaging and image quality, the orthotopic UWF fundus image should clearly show the optic disc, macular area, and vortex veins without iris shadow or lens occlusion. The interference of

Table 7.2.   Statistics of data distribution.

Source	Camera	Location	Patient	Image Total	Normal	Abnormal	RT&RD	DR	Myopia	Cataract	Glaucoma	AMD	AH	MF
PE	PT 200x	North–West	1379	1512	1010	502	0	0	62	32	29	45	17	8
SP	Donate	North–West	220	446	241	205	17	25	163	0	0	0	0	0
ZS	PT 200x	South–East	331	686	144	542	402	81	59	0	0	0	0	0
Total			1930	2644	1395	1249	419	106	284	32	29	45	17	8

Notes: Location: the regional distribution of the cooperative hospitals above in China. Camera : models of Optos cameras available currently.

eyelids and eyelashes on imaging results should be minimized and the coverage should be less than 10 times the visual field. However, we observe a range of imaging noise in the UWF images, caused by such factors as camera dust, blurred lens, or insufficient light, as shown in Fig. 7.1(b). Besides, the areas of different lesions are often very different, and some small lesions may only occupy dozens of pixels, which cannot be accurately identified in the poor photographs.

Therefore, some preprocessing is necessary, and six methods (histogram equalization (HE), adaptive histogram equalization (AHE) (Stark, 2000), intensity rescaling, gamma correction, sigmoid adjustment, and limited contrast AHE (CLAHE)) are empirically explored to improve the quality of the original training images.

First, HE is used to improve the overall brightness of the images and reveal hidden information at the edges of the retina images. However, certain parts of images processed via HE may appear extremely bright, whereas others may appear extremely dim with blurry details. Based on the principle of block processing, AHE is adopted to improve local contrast and enhance edge definition in each image region.

To extract the features from the overall dark image, a contrast stretching algorithm is introduced to readjust the contrast range of the meta-pixels to make it more even. Pixel values less than the minimum are set to 0, whereas those greater than the maximum are set to 255.

If a large number of gray pixel values or a range of lower gray areas are assigned the same value, the image information is lost. However, storing these similar gray values in a higher-level area wastes storage space. In view of this problem, we use gamma correction: the range of the image's pixel strength is adjusted from (0,255) to (0,1.0), and the gamma value is adjusted to 0.45 so that the image details could be clearly displayed in the low-gray areas.

For gamut mapping tasks, brightness reproduction of the mapping image plays an important role in the quality of the final image, and the key is to maintain the perceived brightness contrast of the original image. The sigmoid function is a feasible solution to this problem, as it can not only enhance the image's contrast in a limited dynamic range but also compress the details of highlights and shadows.

Although the aforementioned local contrast method can enhance images' visual interpretability to a great extent, it can still distort

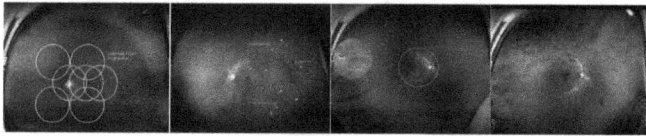

(a) Typical cases

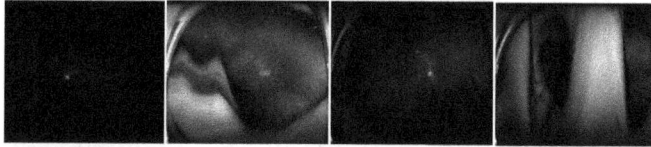

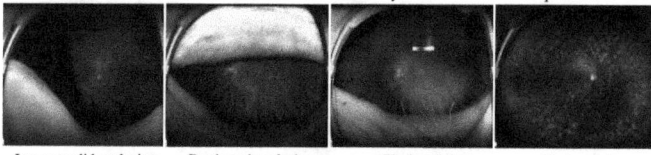

Underexposure   Dusty   Eyelash   Disqualification

Lower eyelid occlusion   Ptosis and eyelash   Flash and dust   Postoperative

(b) Poor quality images

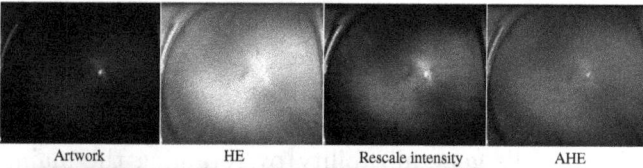

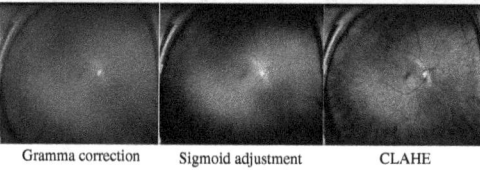

Artwork   HE   Rescale intensity   AHE

Gramma correction   Sigmoid adjustment   CLAHE

(c) Image preprocessing methods

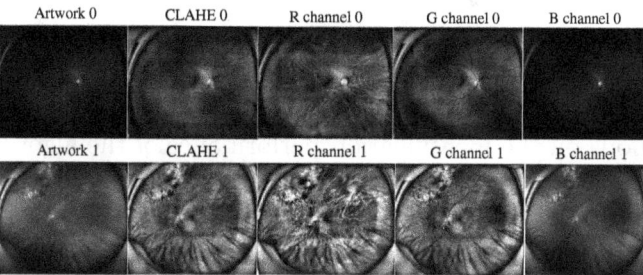

Artwork 0   CLAHE 0   R channel 0   G channel 0   B channel 0

Artwork 1   CLAHE 1   R channel 1   G channel 1   B channel 1

(d) Two images via CLAHE preprocessing

Fig. 7.1.   Examples of the dataset. In (d), Artwork 0 is a normal image and Artwork 1 is an abnormal image. R channel is helpful to show deep structures such as choroid, while G and B channels are useful for shallow structures.

the images due to an excessive increase in local contrast. To make the local details in the darker or lighter areas around the macula and optic papilla as strong and clear as possible, we use CLAHE with a contrast threshold (clipLimit = 5.0) to remove the noise effects generated by non-image parts (Zuiderveld, 1994). Figure 7.1(c) shows the visual comparison before and after all the above image preprocessing for a UWF image. Figure 7.1(d) illustrates in detail the use of the CLAHE method to show the distribution of fundus characteristics in the retinal and choroid layers of two UWF images (normal and abnormal). These characteristics of different granularity of the same spatial location obtained by layering are all fused into the network input, which provide a reliable diagnostic basis for the identification of fundus abnormalities.

7.3.5   *Data augmentation*

Given the limited training dataset, we adopt seven data augmentation techniques, including data normalization, random scaling (0.2), random horizontal or vertical flips (0.2), horizontal or vertical shift (0.2), and random rotation by $0° - 40°$. Meanwhile, the processes help improve the model's generalizability by retaining the main features of the original images rather than accurately copying the images.

7.4   Model and Methodology

7.4.1   *Aim and objective*

The following two aims motivate this study in this work:

(1) to experimentally explore the impact of the images preprocess methods on the identification performance of the algorithms for fundus anomalies and to further develop an early abnormal fundus screening system,

(2) to explore the impact of the preprocess methods on the diagnostic performance of the algorithms for the three fundus diseases including RT&RD, DR, and myopia and to further develop an automatic diagnostic system for three fundus diseases.

7.4.2 Strategy and framework

In this study, 'algorithm', 'learner', 'basic learner', and 'component' refer to an independent neural network used in an ensemble.

Each system consists of two learning layers: the first is a basic learning layer composed of some independent basic learners, and the second layer is a meta-learner that combines these learners and corrects the deviations between them. Every basic learner is a two-stage neural network: the first stage is a feature extractor to represent high-level features at different semantic levels directly from UWF images, and the second stage is a customized classifier that makes the final predictions based on the diverse features. Moreover, the ensemble method of weighted stacking does not require considerable components and is suitable for parallel processing between components (Ting and Witten, 1999), thus it is ideal in the study.

7.4.3 Selection of feature extractors

Generally, a larger convolution kernel is preferred for images with more global information distribution, while a smaller convolution kernel is preferred for images with more local information distribution. In this study, important information about peripheral retinopathy tends to be scattered throughout the edges of UWF images, which makes it more difficult for a single feature extractor to select an appropriate convolution kernel size.

To solve this problem, the InceptionV3 network is ideal to be used as a feature extractor in the bottom part of a component, as it can not only flexibly fuse feature maps of different scales but also effectively reduce computational demands. However, larger networks are more prone to vanishing gradient problems. To reduce this tendency, the InceptionResnetV2 network (which combines the advantages of the ResNet and Inception Network architectures) is selected as the second feature extractor. Similarly, Xception is chosen as the third feature extractor because it can improve the InceptionV3 model without increasing network complexity. Comparative experiments with the other two pretraining models (DesNet201 and Resnet50) are applied for objectivity. The results demonstrated that the series of Inception methods are more effective in our study (Table 7.3).

Table 7.3. Metrics of the basic learners of the screening system(%)

Method	Model	Accuracy	Sensitivity	Specificity	Precision	Kappa	F1_score	Youden
Baseline	ResNet50	88.43	80.00	96.67	89.47	88.33	88.33	76.67
	DenseNet201	87.71	85.36	90.00	87.77	75.40	87.69	75.36
0: No pretreatment	InceptionV3	89.88	81.95	97.62	90.91	79.72	89.81	79.57
	Xception	90.84	82.44	99.05	92.04	81.65	90.77	81.49
	InceptionResnetV2	**90.12**	**83.90**	**96.19**	**90.76**	**80.21**	**90.08**	**80.09**
	Ensemble	90.36	82.44	98.10	91.41	80.68	90.29	80.53
1: HE	**InceptionV3**	**91.08**	**88.29**	**93.81**	**91.22**	**82.15**	**91.08**	**82.10**
	Xception	91.81	84.88	98.57	92.64	83.59	91.76	83.45
	InceptionResnetV2	92.53	86.34	98.57	93.21	85.04	92.50	84.91
2: Rescal	InceptionV3	91.57	84.39	98.57	92.45	83.10	91.52	82.96
	Xception	90.36	86.34	94.29	90.63	80.70	90.34	80.63
	InceptionResnetV2	**91.81**	**91.22**	**92.38**	**91.81**	**83.61**	**91.81**	**83.60**
3: AHE	**InceptionV3**	**93.01**	**90.73**	**95.24**	**93.11**	**86.01**	**93.01**	**85.97**
	Xception	91.08	85.85	96.19	91.55	82.14	91.06	82.04
	InceptionResnetV2	90.60	82.93	98.10	91.59	81.17	90.54	81.02

4: Gamma correction	InceptionV3	92.29	88.29	96.19	92.57	84.56	92.27	84.48
	Xception	**92.29**	**90.73**	**93.81**	**92.34**	**84.57**	**92.29**	**84.54**
	InceptionResnetV2	91.57	87.32	95.71	91.88	83.11	91.55	83.03
5: Sigmoid	InceptionV3	90.84	81.46	93.33	90.96	81.67	90.84	81.63
	Xception	91.57	84.88	98.10	92.34	83.10	91.52	82.97
	InceptionResnetV2	**91.57**	**90.24**	**92.86**	**91.60**	**83.13**	**91.56**	**83.10**
6: CLAHE	InceptionV3	92.77	90.24	95.24	92.89	85.53	92.76	85.48
	Xception	92.05	88.29	95.71	92.30	84.08	92.03	84.01
	InceptionResnetV2	**93.73**	**91.22**	**96.19**	**93.86**	**87.46**	**93.73**	**87.41**

Notes: InceptionResnetV2: one basic learner named InceptionResnetV2, which takes InceptionResnetV2 pretraining model as inner feature extractor. The bold terms indicate the best model and the related values of each performance index.

7.4.4   *Design of customized classifiers*

Two customized neural networks, a deep convolutional neural network (DCNN) and a deep full connection network (DFNN), are designed as alternative classifiers for the feature extractors in the systems.

(1) For the DCNN, the output from one feature extractor (with the original top-level removed) is convolved using two custom 3×3 convolution blocks to further reduce dimensions. However, one main issue arising from the aforementioned feature extraction is that the error of the convolutional layer's parameters causes deviation of the estimated means. Max-pooling is ideal to address this problem because it can reduce this error and retain more texture information (Boureau *et al.*, 2010). Therefore, each convolutional block is designed to include a 2×2 maximum pooling layer with a rectified linear unit (Relu) functional layer to improve the model's performance. The Relu layer is followed by two fully connected layers with 1024 and 512 hidden neurons, respectively, and the dropout strategy is adopted for regularization ($p = 0.25$) after each of the above layers (Stark and Fitzgerald, 1994).

(2) For the DFNN, different from the max-pooling strategy adopted in the DCNN, we deploy a global average pooling (GAP) layer to retain the spatial information extracted by the convolution and pooling layers of its feature extractor. The GAP layer further averages all pixels of each feature map and outputs the average value to reduce the total number of parameters in the network and minimize overfitting. The GAP layer is followed by four fully connected layers with 2048, 1024, 512, and 256 hidden neurons, respectively. Leaky Relu layers and dropout layers ($p = 0.2$) are added after each dense layer above.

The final layers of the classifiers above are standard softmax layers used to regularize weights for network calculations with binary cross-entropy as a loss function for the screening system or with cross-entropy served for the diagnosis system. The cross-entropies can reveal the distance or degree of closeness between the true labels and the predicted values. Figure 7.3(b) shows the two customized classifiers' structures of the screening system.

7.4.5 *Performance metrics*

Several metrics are used to evaluate the performance of models from reliability and effectiveness. Accuracy intuitively represents the proportion of samples with correct classifications. Precision is the ratio of correctly predicted positive samples, and it is especially relevant in problems with severe class imbalance. Sensitivity is the safety standard for patients in the screening system and specificity affects the number of patients who need to be referred to. Kappa measures the degree of reliability obtained by repeated tests under the same conditions. A receiver operating characteristic curve (ROC) with a corresponding AUC value can graphically represent the balance between sensitivity and specificity. In cases of extreme imbalance, the F1_score (which is the harmonic average of precision and sensitivity) should be considered. F_β is the weighted harmonic average of the F1_score. The purpose of the Youden index (Youden) is to verify the entire model's diagnostic authenticity.

7.5 Experiments

7.5.1 *Experimental setup*

All algorithms are implemented via Keras and performed on an Intel Xeon E5-2620 CPU and NVIDIA Tesla K40 GPU in parallel and independently. Images are scaled into 299×299 or 224×224 to reduce the computational cost. Six independent preprocessing subsets are respectively added to the training dataset of the systems; therefore, each training subset consists of three parts: the original data, the data generated by the preprocessing method, and the data augmentation of the first two.

Basic learners use a mini-bach of 5 or 8 images for training. RMSprop is used as an optimizer in the screening system with an initial learning rate of 2e-5. SGD is used for optimization in the diagnosis system with a basic learning rate of 0.01 and a momentum of 0.9. The learning rates would be reduced to 2e-10 with a constant step size of 0.1; and network training could be interrupted by EarlyStopping after 10 complete passes if the loss on the validation set is no longer dropping.

7.5.2 Screening system

The PE dataset is divided into three parts: training, tuning, and testing at 7:2:1, where each subset is case-related. The SP dataset and the ZS dataset are used for clinical validation.

7.5.2.1 System design

A group of basic learners with better classification effects is obtained by connecting the extractors (InceptionV3 and InceptionResnetV2) to DCNN, and the Xception extractor to DFNN. The learners are assigned the same names as their internal pretraining extractors for convenience. Generally, the screening system consists of three component pools: first, a pool C0 named "Xception" and a pool C1 named "InceptionResnetV2" are combined via weight coefficients of 0.51 and 0.49, and then further integrated with a pool C3 named "InceptionV3" with weight coefficients of 0.48 and 0.52. The Gamma-based learner is taken as the 'Xception' pool due to its highest sensitivity compared with other pretreatment learners. For the InceptionResnetV2 pool, we first averagely integrate three InceptionResnetV2 learners trained by Rescal, Sigmoid, and CLAHE image preprocessing methods, and then further combine the integrated model with the CLAHE-based InceptionResnetV2 learner with weight coefficients of 0.49 and 0.51, respectively. The InceptionV3 pool is obtained by the weighted average of two basic learners trained under AHE and CLAHE preprocessing. Figure 7.2 shows the system framework.

7.5.2.2 Analysis of empirical

Compared with the non-preprocessing methods, the results indicate that the preprocessing methods may be useful to improve the models' learning efficiency (Table 7.3). For example, without image optimization, the Xception pool performs poorly in the trade-off between its sensitivity and specificity (82.44% and 99.05%); in the Gamma correction method, however, the sensitivity is significantly improved and the trade-off with the specificity remained at a good level (90.73% and 93.81%). In the AHE method, the InceptionV3 pool significantly increases its sensitivity from 81.95% to 90.73%, whereas the specificity drops only from 97.62% to 95.24%. In the CLAHE method, the InceptionResnetV2 pool increases its sensitivity from 83.90% to 91.22% while maintaining a constant specificity of 96.19%. Table 7.4

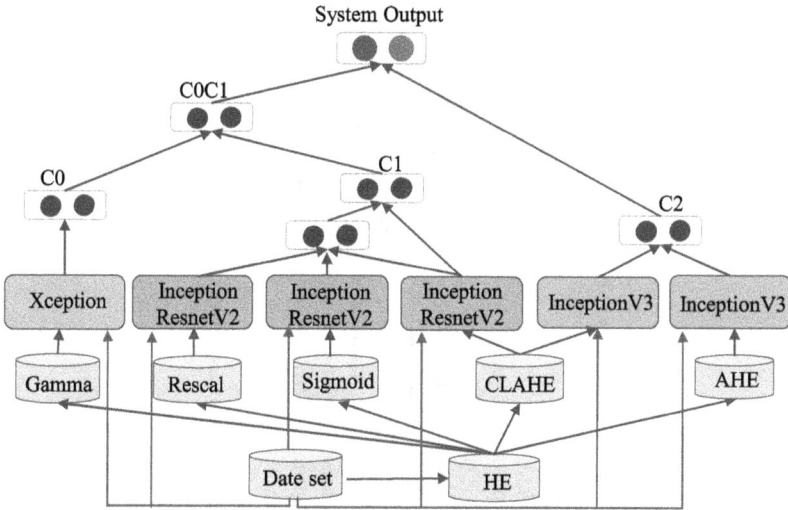

(a) Method

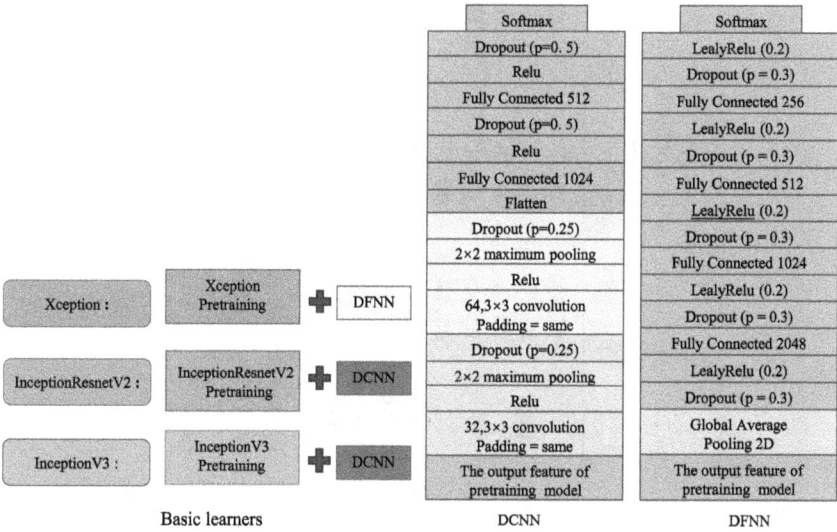

(b) Three components

Fig. 7.2.   The fundus screening system. Each basic learner uses different algorithms to represent knowledge and different learning deviations based on the various preprocessed data and explores the hypothesis space from multiple dimensions, thereby generating different classifier pools. Therefore, when their predictions are combined, the ensemble model is more accurate than each member. Moreover, the fusion of class probabilities and the weighted strategy are essential for the successful application of stacking in this classification task.

Table 7.4. Metrics of the component pools of the screening system (%).

Model	Accuracy	Sensitivity	Specificity	Precision	Kappa	F1.score	Youden
C0: Xception pool	92.29	90.73	93.81	92.34	84.57	92.29	84.54
C1: InceptionResnetV2 pool	93.74	90.73	96.67	93.91	87.46	93.73	87.40
C0C1	93.49	88.78	98.10	93.90	86.97	93.48	86.88
C2: InceptionV3 pool	93.98	91.71	96.19	94.08	87.94	93.97	87.90
System Output	**95.42**	**93.17**	**97.62**	**95.53**	**90.84**	**95.42**	**90.79**

Notes: C0 represents the Xception pool obtained by one Xception learner trained based on the original images and the Gamma image preprocessing method. C1 is the InceptionResnetV2 pool obtained by three InceptionResnetV2 learners trained based on the original images and three image preprocessing methods: Rescal, Sigmoid, and CLAHE, respectively. C2 refers to the InceptionV3 pool obtained by two InceptionV3 learners trained based on the original images and two image preprocessing methods: CLAHE and AHE, respectively. C0C1 means the ensemble of the above two pools: Xception pool and InceptionResnetV2 pool. "System Output" represents the ensemble model of C0C1 and C2. The bold terms indicate the best model and the related values of each performance index.

Table 7.5.   Metrics of the screening system on three test sets.

Source	Data scale	Accuracy	Sensitivity	Specificity	Precision	Kappa	F1_score	Youden
PE	415	95.42	93.17	97.62	95.53	90.84	95.42	90.79
SP	446	90.36	91.73	88.89	90.39	80.68	90.35	80.62
ZS	686	90.96	91.32	89.58	90.96	74.81	91.27	80.91

shows that the sensitivity of the system is significantly improved by 10.73% (from 82.44% to 93.17%), and the specificity is slightly reduced by 0.48% (from 98.10% to 97.62%).

7.5.2.3   *Generalization performance*

Table 7.5 indicates that the sensitivity and specificity of the screening system to the SP dataset are 91.73% and 88.89%, and to the ZS dataset are 91.32% and 89.58%. Although the performance of the system on the two test datasets declines, it still maintains some generalization. The main reasons may be as follows: (1) the number of abnormal fundus images of SP and ZS is much more than that of the PE training set; (2) the limited training set, the difference between different cameras, and the difference between UWF photographers all affect the system performance. Therefore, if more data from different sources could be added to the training process of the screening system, the system generalization might be improved.

7.5.3   *Diagnostic system*

7.5.3.1   *Data partition*

The SP dataset, the ZS dataset, and the images labeled as "normal" or "myopia" of the PE dataset together constitute the dataset of the four diseases, which includes 1,395 normal images and 809 disease images labeled as one of the three categories "RT&RD", "DR", or "myopia". The disease dataset is divided into a training set, test set, and validation set at the ratio of 7:2:1.

7.5.3.2   *System design*

The above three extractors (InceptionV3, InceptionResNetV2, and Xception) are used in the experiments; and compared with the

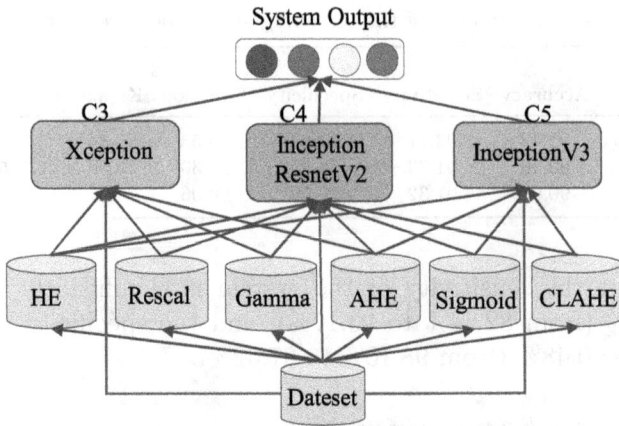

(a) Method

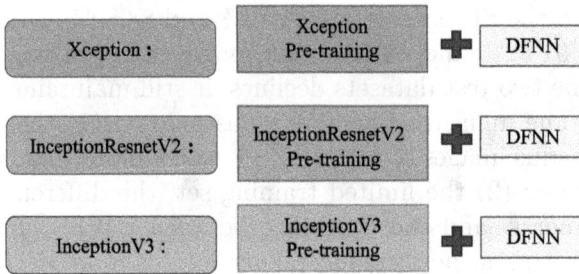

(b) Three components

Fig. 7.3.   The disease diagnosis system. C3 represents the Xception pool obtained by four Xception learners trained based on the original images and four image preprocessing methods, respectively: HE, Rescal, Gamma, and AHE. C4 is the InceptionResnetV2 pool obtained by the original images and six InceptionResnetV2 learners trained based on six image preprocessing methods, respectively. C5 refers to the InceptionV3 pool obtained by the original images and four InceptionV3 learners trained based on four image preprocessing methods: HE, AHE, Sigmoid, and CLAHE, respectively. "System output" means the ensemble model of C3, C4, and C5.

classifier DCNN, learners embedded with DFNN work better in the experiments. Sequentially, the impacts of the six different preprocessing methods on the diagnosis performance of the algorithms for three fundus diseases are tried, respectively. The outstanding basic learners are finally combined into three algorithm pools: C3, C4, and C5 (see Fig. 7.3) and further determine the final ensemble framework of the diagnostic system by averaging their softmax scores. The disease diagnostic system is implemented as shown in Fig. 7.3. Comparative experiments without the preprocessing methods are applied for objectivity.

7.5.3.3 *Analysis of empirical*

From Table 7.6, the algorithms have relatively lower sensitivity and high specificity without these preprocessing methods. We think there are two main reasons: first, the limited number of diseases, which constitute respectively only 19%, 4.8%, and 12.9% of the disease dataset; second, the dark color of the parts in the original images, which is not conducive to learners' recognition of abnormal signs in these parts.

However, with the preprocessing methods, the algorithms achieve better average accuracies. For example, Gamma preprocessing can significantly improve the diagnostic accuracy of the algorithms to RT&RD, some images of which are misdiagnosed as DR. We observe that the main reason is that RT&RD is a complication of DR. CLAHE improves the diagnostic accuracy to myopia well, but images of high myopia are easily misclassified as normal. We check the images and find that the main reason is the limited training images of myopia and the pathological characteristics of high myopia images are not obvious. The sensitivity of the algorithms to DR is increased by nearly 12% under Gamma. The DR images are misdiagnosed primarily as RT&RD, and the main reason for this phenomenon is that the models cannot fully learn the characteristics of DR. Finally, the diagnose system achieves an accuracy of 97.45%, and Table 7.7 shows more details about the classification reports of the three diseases.

7.6 Discussion

7.6.1 *Image optimization*

The contrast of UWF images used in the study is low, which seriously limits the extraction of fine features on UWF images by the depth model. Therefore, the high specificity and low sensitivity of prediction results have always been the problems of this project. By adjusting the contrast, brightness, and gray level of the images, and

Table 7.6. Metrics of the learners of the disease diagnose system (%).

Method	Model	Accuracy	Sensitivity (± standard deviation)				F1_score (± standard deviation)				Youden
			Normal	RT&RD	DR	Myopia	Normal	RT&RD	DR	Myopia	
0: No pretreatment	IncepRes	91.43(1.62)	97.00(0.82)	82.67(4.50)	68.33(1.89)	83.67(0.94)	97.00(0.82)	86.50(3.50)	69.00(2.16)	76.33(6.01)	89.86(3.10)
	Xception	93.35(0.87)	97.75(0.43)	88.25(1.79)	75.00(7.11)	80.75(1.30)	97.25(0.43)	90.75(2.16)	75.75(4.92)	80.50(0.87)	91.15(0.75)
	Incepv3	92.90(0.47)	97.67(0.47)	87.67(1.70)	71.33(3.68)	80.00(0.00)	97.00(0.00)	89.67(0.00)	73.00(1.24)	80.00(1.40)	90.83(0.60)
1: HE	IncepRes	96.18(0.35)	98.50(0.50)	94.50(1.50)	85.50(4.50)	88.00(5.00)	98.50(0.50)	95.00(1.00)	82.50(3.50)	88.50(1.50)	95.53(0.01)
	Xception	95.91(0.61)	98.33(0.47)	95.33(0.47)	77.67(4.71)	87.67(2.05)	98.67(0.47)	94.67(1.24)	80.33(2.94)	88.67(0.94)	95.97(0.59)
	Incepv3	96.12(0.68)	98.00(0.00)	96.75(1.92)	76.00(6.12)	89.50(3.64)	98.25(0.5)	94.75(1.78)	79.50(3.77)	86.75(2.12)	95.43(1.01)
2: Rescal	IncepRes	96.07(0.37)	98.50(0.50)	94.25(1.30)	81.00(3.54)	90.25(3.27)	98.75(0.43)	95.00(0.71)	83.00(1.87)	87.00(1.58)	96.12(0.98)
	Xception	95.49(0.47)	98.25(0.83)	94.50(1.11)	79.50(6.06)	85.75(4.65)	98.25(0.43)	95.50(0.86)	81.00(4.12)	83.50(3.04)	94.83(1.21)
	Incepv3	96.37(0.55)	99.00(0.87)	93.33(0.83)	82.67(4.33)	92.67(2.92)	98.33(0.43)	95.00(1.12)	82.67(5.55)	90.00(0.83)	96.10(1.34)
3: AHE	IncepRes	95.83(0.36)	98.61(0.48)	95.30(0.82)	78.50(5.09)	87.80(3.27)	98.30(0.43)	94.75(0.43)	81.50(4.15)	88.00(1.22)	95.00(1.14)
	Xception	95.20(0.09)	98.50(0.50)	93.50(1.50)	78.50(5.59)	84.50(4.60)	98.00(0.00)	94.25(0.43)	76.50(1.12)	86.00(0.71)	94.14(1.24)
	Incepv3	95.97(0.34)	98.00(0.71)	93.50(0.50)	81.00(3.53)	94.30(2.16)	98.8(0.43)	94.3(0.83)	83.00(2.50)	90.30(1.90)	96.40(0.79)
4: Gamma correction	IncepRes	95.37(0.37)	97.67(0.47)	95.33(0.47)	81.00(2.50)	89.67(2.87)	98.30(0.00)	95.00(0.00)	81.67(3.09)	85.67(1.7)	94.22(1.37)
	Xception	95.91(0.61)	98.67(0.47)	95.67(0.47)	88.67(1.89)	81.33(3.86)	98.33(0.47)	95.67(0.47)	84.67(0.94)	85.67(2.49)	94.38(1.80)
	Incepv3	95.91(0.47)	98.33(0.47)	95.67(2.05)	84.00(4.24)	86.00(2.94)	98.0(0.00)	94.33(0.94)	86.67(1.70)	88.33(2.05)	93.92(0.98)
5: Sigmoid	IncepRes	96.41(0.66)	98.50(0.87)	94.25(0.43)	89.25(6.02)	92.25(2.59)	98.75(0.43)	94.75(1.09)	83.25(2.68)	90.25(3.90)	97.14(1.15)
	Xception	95.89(0.34)	98.50(0.50)	94.50(0.87)	79.75(4.14)	87.75(3.96)	98.75(0.43)	95.00(0.71)	77.50(4.03)	87.25(1.78)	96.13(0.87)
	Incepv3	95.75(0.26)	97.75(0.43)	94.50(1.11)	82.00(5.04)	91.50(4.71)	98.00(0.00)	93.75(0.83)	83.00(2.55)	89.00(1.87)	95.08(0.78)
6: CLAHE	IncepRes	95.83(0.32)	9800(0.00)	93.50(0.5)	83.50(2.50)	90.50(2.05)	98.00(0.00)	94.50(0.50)	79.50(0.50)	89.50(0.52)	95.17(0.34)
	Xception	95.60(0.28)	98.25(0.00)	95.75(1.24)	75.25(6.6)	90.33(3.77)	98.33(0.50)	94.67(0.50)	79.00(0.50)	85.67(0.00)	94.59(0.54)
	Incepv3	95.60(0.37)	98.33(0.47)	93.00(2.45)	74.33(4.71)	92.00(1.41)	98.33(0.47)	94.33(1.24)	77.67(4.99)	87.00(0.81)	95.63(0.15)

Table 7.7. Metrics of the component pools of the disease diagnosis system (%).

Model	Accuracy	Sensitivity				Fl_score				Youden
		Normal	RT&RD	DR	Myopia	Normal	RT&RD	DR	Myopia	
C3: Xception pool	96.75	99	96	90	85	99	96	84	89	96.90
C4: Inception-ResnetV2 pool	96.52	99	96	81	90	98	95	85	91	95.18
C5: Inception V3 pool	96.53	99	97	79	90	99	97	80	88	96.54
System Output	**97.45**	**99**	**98**	**86**	**93**	**99**	**97**	**88**	**92**	**97.58**

highlighting the features of the lesions and diseases, the image optimization methods may be helpful to improve the prediction ability of the models in the study.

Besides, based on specific datasets, different algorithms have different prediction capabilities for each preprocessing method. Gamma correction makes gray images clearer and lesions more prominent, which indicates to be more conducive to improve the learning ability of the Xception network. When CLAHE and AHE improve the local contrasts and edge definitions of each area of the images, it also significantly improves the learning ability of the Inceptionv3 learner for fundus lesion features. Similarly, the prediction performance of InceptionResnetV2 networks is also improved after the contrast and brightness adjustment of images by Rescal, Sigmoid, and CLAHE, respectively.

Despite the preprocessing methods in research sometimes reducing the available signals indiscriminately, the images generated by them retain the main features from their original images in most cases. Besides, this method ensures the expansion of the training set, while the image is not completely copied.

7.6.2 *Medical implication*

China has one of the largest numbers of blind and visually impaired patients in the world; therefore, fundus health screening is the first line of defense for early prevention of fundus diseases and protection of fundus health. In this study, the diversity of fundus information in the dataset helps heterogeneous populations to participate more easily in screening efforts for fundus abnormalities.

Moreover, the performance of retinal disease screening is an extremely urgent task. RT&RD treatment and prevention are cost-effective when compared to other retinal diseases. DR patients are 25-fold more likely to develop blindness. The myopia rate in China is 10% higher than the world average. Therefore, DeepUWF helps inspectors to assess the risk of disease in the general public and enhance the feasibility of evaluation.

7.6.3 *Limitations*

We have to admit that the labeling work is based on the clinical experience of the ophthalmologist, so when there are subtle signs or symptoms that most clinicians can't identify in the images used, the algorithm can have different performances. Moreover, the gradient disappearance in deep learning makes the system tend to be one of the local optimum solutions. Besides, the heterogeneity of datasets in different hospitals, the differences in acquisition equipment, and the differences in imaging parameters are the main reasons that affect the generalization performance of the system.

7.6.4 *Future work*

Therefore, in the follow-up work, we will collect more data from different hospitals, conduct multi-center data joint learning, learn various representative medical characteristics, and effectively improve the actual performance of the system. Moreover, multi-pathological-signs detection and multi-diseases diagnosis will be carried out to provide more accurate and effective clinical assistance.

7.7 Conclusion

In this study, we establish a UWF imaging medical dataset and design two customized classifiers. By combining these classifiers with advanced pretraining models, we further develop an automatic fundus health screening system called DeepUWF, which includes an abnormal fundus screening subsystem and a disease diagnosis subsystem. To make the depth model more effective in extracting the fine features of UWF images, we study the impact of six different image preprocessing methods on the models' prediction performance. The experimental results show that the preprocessing method based on specific datasets can improve the prediction sensitivity of the model and maintain its stable specificity. Without ophthalmologists, DeepUWF has potential application value for fundus health screening and workflow improvement.

Chapter 8

DeepUWF-Plus: Automatic Fundus Identification and Diagnosis System Based on Ultrawide-field Fundus Imaging

Poor eye health is a major public health problem, and the timely detection and diagnosis of fundus abnormalities are important for eye health protection. Traditional imaging models can hinder the comprehensive evaluation of fundus abnormalities due to the use of a narrow field of view. The emerging ultrawide-field (UWF) imaging model surpasses this limitation in a non-invasive, wide-view manner and is suitable for fundus observation and screening. Nevertheless, manual screening is labor-intensive and subjective, especially in the absence of an ophthalmologist. Therefore, a set of auxiliary screening methods for a fundus screening service using a combination of deep learning and UWF imaging technology, which is designated as DeepUWF-Plus, are proposed. This service includes a subsystem for the screening of fundus, a subsystem for the identification of abnormalities regarding four important fundus locations, and a subsystem for the diagnosis of four retinal diseases that threaten vision. The influence of two-stage and one-stage classification strategies on the prediction performance of the model is experimentally investigated to alleviate severe class imbalance and similarity between classes, and evaluate the effectiveness and reliability of the system. Our experimental results show that DeepUWF-Plus is effective when using the two-stage strategy, especially for identifying signs or symptoms of minor diseases. DeepUWF-Plus can improve the practicality of fundus screening and enable ophthalmologists to provide more comprehensive fundus assessments.

8.1   Related Works

8.1.1   *Deep learning with traditional imaging technology*

DL technology is receiving increasing attention in the field of ophthalmology. Currently, major eye diseases that can be screened with DL technology include DR, age-related macular degeneration (AMD), and glaucoma (Abràmoff *et al.*, 2016; Ting *et al.*, 2017; Zhang *et al.*, 2019; Burlina *et al.*, 2017; Raghavendra *et al.*, 2018; Asaoka *et al.*, 2016). These DL algorithms reportedly have diagnostic capabilities similar to those of retinal experts and have achieved landmark results (Topol, 2019). However, the accuracy of eye disease screening depends on the degree of insight into the entire fundus, including peripheral retina and vascular pathology. Most studies have employed traditional fundus imaging (e.g., color fundus imaging), which provides minimal information regarding the peripheral retina due to the narrow field of view and is likely to cause missed diagnosis.

8.1.2   *Deep learning with emerging UWF imaging technology*

UWF imaging can be used to overcome the above visual field limitations and provide a more comprehensive, intuitive assessment of patients' fundus abnormalities. Thus far, DL-based UWF imaging analysis has shown impressive performance in retinal diseases, providing new ideas for the implementation of various fundus screening and remote ophthalmology programs. Li *et al.* developed a cascaded DL system containing two binary models via InceptionResNetV2 network. The first model was used to identify RD and non-RD based on 10,451 images (2009 RD images) with a sensitivity of 96.1% and a specificity of 99.6%. The second model was used to discern macula-on/off RD further based on the above 1771 RD images with a sensitivity of 93.8% and a specificity of 90.9% (Li *et al.*, 2020).

Matsuba *et al.* developed a DL network to predict exudative AMD with a 100% sensitivity and a 97.31% specificity based on 364 images (AMD:137) (Matsuba *et al.*, 2019). From a practical point of view, several studies showed that the DL models perform better than machine learning by comparing the predictive performance of VGG16 networks with support vector machines (SVM) on branch retinal vein occlusions (446 images), rhegmatogenous RD (831 images), and central retinal vein occlusion (363 images) (Ohsugi *et al.*, 2017; Nagasato *et al.*, 2019, 2018).

However, these studies have several evident shortcomings. First, an important limitation of many current DL algorithms is their binary nature, whereby these DL models are developed using normal fundus images and abnormal images that depict a single disease. The diversity of eye-related diseases and urgency of referral make this disease-specific strategy often inappropriate for heterogeneous populations enrolled in retinal screening programs (Choi *et al.*, 2017; Fenner *et al.*, 2018). Second, the potential value of image-based neural networks in identifying fundus signs is not considered, which leads to their potential failure to detect clinically substantial diseases (Lynch *et al.*, 2017). Third, most of the studies present results derived from small databases, limiting the generalization and robustness of systems.

By contrast, based on a larger UWF dataset collected from different hospitals (total of 10,541 images, of which 5,014 are lesion images), DL technology was used in this study for the screening of multiple diseases and key parts of the fundus to improve the practicality of fundus screening for large-scale populations.

8.2 Dataset

8.2.1 *Materials*

Between June 2018 and November 2019, 6434 UWF photos of 2434 patients from the Zhongshan Eye Centre (ZS) and 5236 images of 1853 patients from the Sichuan Advanced Medical Examination Centre (PE) were collected. Nearly all patients in ZS had one to six UWF photos per eye, while patients in PE typically had one or two UWF photos per eye.

8.2.2 *Annotation standard*

Based on the latest American Association of Ophthalmology Clinical Guidelines (Bagheri *et al.*, 2016), a UWF image annotation system was developed to obtain high-quality annotation data. In this system, the annotator first evaluates the quality of each fundus image and distinguishes between representations of normal fundus and abnormal fundus. The annotator then marks the type of abnormal signs in the fundus image. The observation of pathological signs includes four important fundus components: optic neuropathy area, retinopathy area, macular lesion region, and vitreous lesion area. The corresponding fundus components are shown in Fig. 8.1.

Generally, each area contains 3–17 symbol subcategories. Finally, the annotator provides specific diagnosis opinions regarding 17 common retinal diseases in China. Table 8.1 shows details of the specific assessment. Figure 8.2 shows the respective sign abnormalities of the four fundus regions and the symptoms of the four diseases in this study. The annotators in this study included one retina specialist with more than 30 years of experience in retinal research and three board-certified ophthalmologists with more than five years of clinical

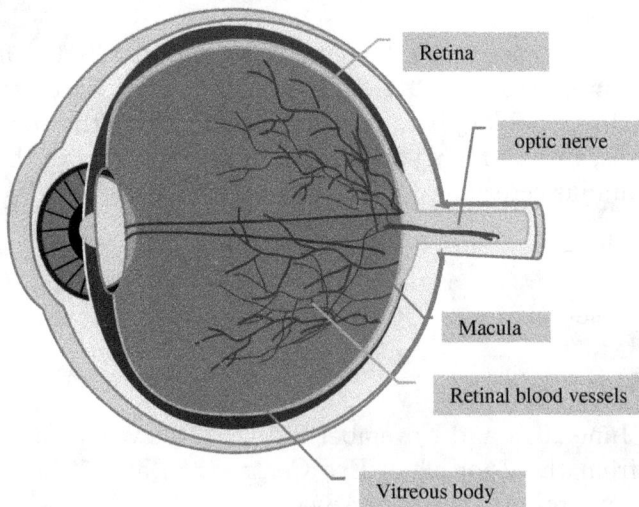

Fig. 8.1.   Eye anatomy.

Table 8.1. Sign and disease annotation details.

Sign Lesion Area	Possible Lesions or Disease Categories
Optic disc lesion	Optic disc atrophy, Blurred optic disc boundary, Optic disc dysplasia, Cup disc ratio increases, Pigmented patches atrophic rings, and Others
Retinopathy	Retinal artery tortuosity, Retinal vein tortuosity, Retinal vascular occlusion or white sheath, Retinal hemorrhage, Retinal exudation, Peripheral retinal degeneration area, RT, Retinal pigmentation (or proliferation), Proliferating membrane, Neovascularization, Peripheral retinal regional abnormal color, Loss of retinal pigment, Retinitis pigmentosa, Yellow-white lesions, RD, and Others
Macular lesion	Macular hemorrhage, Macular exudation, Macular hole, Epimacular membrane, Macular choroidal atrophy, Yellow-white lesions, and Others
Vitreous lesion	Vitreous hemorrhage, Asteroid hyalosis, Vitreous opacity, and Others
Other	Refractive media turbidity, Postoperation, Myelinated nerve fiber, and Others
Fundus disease	DR, Myopia, Cataract, AMD, Glaucoma, RD, RT, Macular edema, Choroid atrophy in macular area, Space occupying lesion, Central retinal vein occlusion (or artery), Vitreous hemorrhage, Papilledema, Optic papilla atrophy, Myelinated nerve fiber, and Others

diagnosis and treatment. The final labeling results were agreed upon by all the annotators, and disagreements were resolved by the senior retina expert.

8.2.3 *Annotation details*

According to the guideline of 'Operation and Reading Specifications of Ultrawide-field Fundus Imaging Technology in China (2018)', when evaluating image quality, the orthographic UWF fundus image should clearly show the optic disc, macular area, and vortex veins without iris shadow or lens occlusion. Therefore, 1462 images with artifacts caused by blinking, closing eyes, and improper shooting positions during shooting were excluded. Moreover, the system was

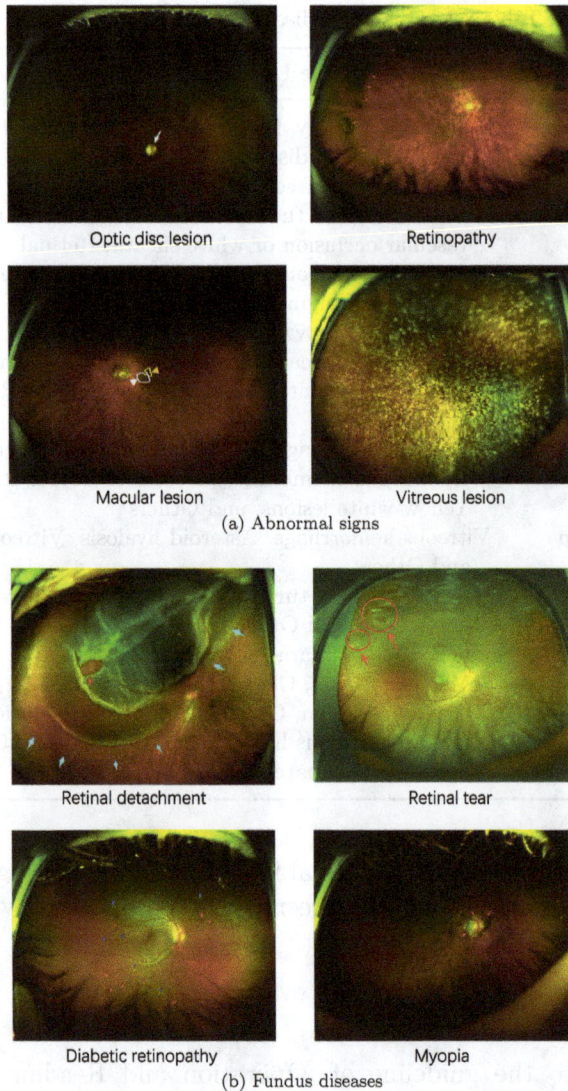

Optic disc lesion

Retinopathy

Macular lesion

Vitreous lesion

(a) Abnormal signs

Retinal detachment

Retinal tear

Diabetic retinopathy

Myopia

(b) Fundus diseases

Fig. 8.2. In (a), the arrow in the upper left indicates a optic nerve atrophy; the arrows in the upper right image indicate retinal lattice degenerations; the yellow arrow in the lower left represents a bleeding and the white arrow represents some gray-white lesions; the lower right is a vitreous asteroid degeneration. In (b), the red arrows in the upper left represent RT, and the blue arrows represent RD; the upper right images show RT; the red arrows in the lower left represent bleeding and the blue arrows represent exudation; the red arrows at the bottom right indicate myopic conus.

designed for the general population, rather than for patients who have already received medical intervention. Therefore, 1431 postoperative images were excluded because they reflected the retinal recovery of the patients. Additionally, images from PE were difficult to assess because of their overall dark color; thus, distinction could only be made between normal and abnormal. Images from ZS were diverse but exhibited an uneven disease distribution. Finally, 8777 screening images, 4541 sign images, and 3429 disease images were obtained. Table 8.2 provides detailed statistics regarding the distribution of images among categories.

8.2.4 *Data preprocessing and augmentation*

The original images were first downsized from 3900×3072 to 299×299 or 224×224 to meet the standard input requirements for pretraining models used in this study. Data were normalized to a range of 0 to 1. Furthermore, data argumentation techniques were adopted to increase the number of images in the training and validation datasets by seven-fold. These techniques included random scaling (0.2), random horizontal and vertical flips (0.2), horizontal and vertical shift (0.2), and random rotation by $0°-40°$. These processes helped increase the diversity of training images and improve the generalization performance of the system. Figure 8.3 shows the details of the split and expansion of the data.

8.3 Model and Methodology

8.3.1 *Aim*

This work was performed to develop three modules: (1) an early automatic fundus screening system, which comprises a binary classification task to judge the presence or absence of an abnormal fundus, (2) an automatic sign part identification system, which comprises a four-class task to predict the areas of fundus abnormal signs, and (3) an automatic disease diagnosis system, which comprises a four-class task to predict the categories of visually threatening retinal diseases.

Table 8.2.　Summary of the four datasets.

Source	Site	M	Pa	Per	Screening			Sign Identification							Disease Diagnosis						
									Sign Category							Disease Category					
					Nor	Abn	S4	Nor	1	2	3	4	s5	S6	Nor	5	6	7	8	s7	S8
Training																					
PE	NT	TX	1482	1~2	2244	297	2541	0	0	0	0	0	0	0	0	0	0	0	0	0	0
ZS	ST	Da	2231	1~6	568	3065	3633	568	404	2464	118	79	3065	3633	575	1526	58	309	275	2168	2743
S0					2812	3362	6174	568	404	2464	118	79	3065	3633	575	1526	58	309	275	2168	2743
Testing																					
PE	NT	TX	371	1~2	1496	199	1695	0	0	0	0	0	0	0	0	0	0	0	0	0	0
ZS	ST	Da	558	1~6	151	757	908	151	91	609	38	19	757	908	144	390	12	81	59	542	686
S1					1647	956	2603	151	91	609	38	19	757	908	144	390	12	81	59	542	686
S2					4459	4318	8777	719	495	3073	156	98	3822	4541	719	1916	70	390	334	2710	3429
The other two testing sets																					
SC	NT	TX	98	1~6	216	205	421	216	55	30	10	4	99	315	216	12	5	25	163	205	421
MY	NT	Da	327	1~5	852	491	1343	852	25	161	25	3	214	1066	852	38	7	80	366	491	1343
S3			5607		5527	5014	10541	1787	575	3264	191	105	4135	5922	1787	1966	82	495	863	3406	5193

Notes: Site: the regional distribution of the cooperative hospitals in China, Pa: the number of patients, ST: Southeast of China. NT: Northwest of China. Nor: Normal. Abn: Abnormal, M: models of optos cameras. Da: Daytona. TX: 200TX. Per: number of fundus photographs taken per eye, 1: optic disc lesion. 2: retinopathy. 3: macular lesions. 4: vitreous lesion, 5: RD. 6: RT. 7: DR. 8: myopia, S0: the sum of images in the training set, S1: the sum of images in the testing set, S2: the sum of images in S0 and S1, S3: the sum of images in S2, SC, and MY, S4: the sum of images in the screening system under different datasets, S5: the sum of lesion images in the sign identification system under different datasets, S6: the sum of images in the sign identification system under different datasets, S7: the sum of lesion images in the diagnosis system under different datasets, S8: the sum of images in the diagnosis system under different datasets.

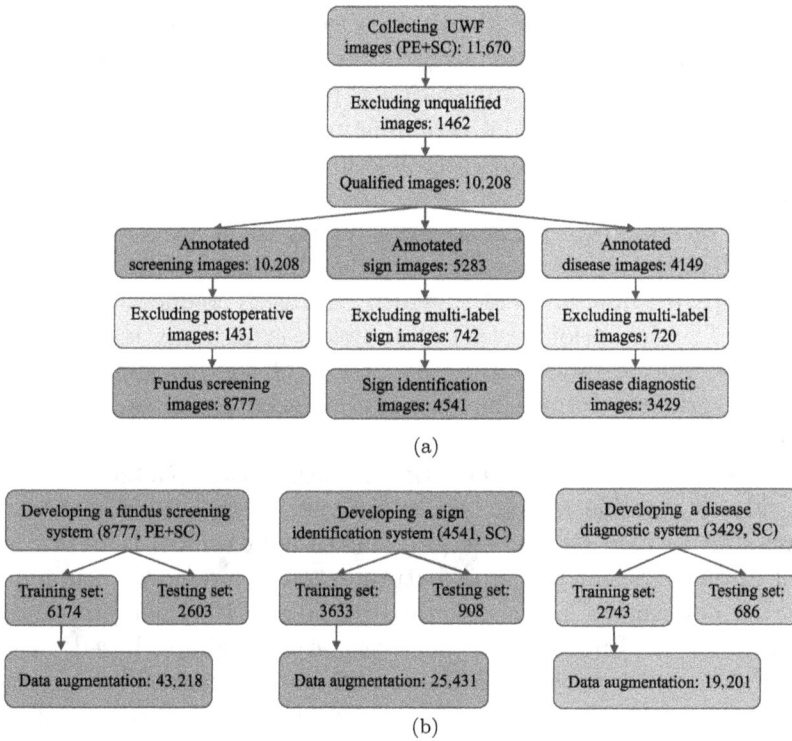

(a)

(b)

Fig. 8.3. The data workflow of the system. (a) Shows the details of data annotation and division and (b) shows data processing during the system development.

Every basic learner of these systems was composed of a feature extractor and a classifier. The feature extractor used one pretraining model, while the classifier was customized in this study. For ease of description, each learner had the same name as its internal feature extractor. Moreover, weighted stacking technology was used to combine multiple models into a higher-quality classifier, thereby achieving better prediction performance. When determining the numbers and identities of base classifiers in the final integration, the only criterion was whether the candidate could improve ensemble performance.

8.3.2 *Feature extractors*

In this study, important information regarding peripheral retinopathy was often scattered on the edges of fundus images. This considerable difference in information location caused a single feature extractor to experience difficulty in selecting an appropriate convolution kernel size. Additionally, the limited availability of training data hindered the direct application of ordinary networks to medical imaging. Thus, a powerful pretraining model must be selected as feature extractor, rather than designing an ordinary deep network from scratch.

The InceptionV3 network may be an ideal feature extractor in this study due to advances in the flexible fusion of the feature maps of different scales, which effectively reduce the computation. The InceptionRestnetv2 network is also an ideal feature extractor that combines the advantages of Resnet and Inception networks, thereby improving classification accuracy. Xception constitutes another improvement to InceptionV3, which can improve the model without increasing network complexity. DenseNet201 was also considered suitable for our study because it can fully use the features and further reduce the gradient disappearance. It performed well in our experiments. The feature extractors remove their inherent full connection layers and then initialize with their pretraining weights on the ImageNet, respectively. After training based on the UWF data, these powerful CNNs of different architecture can extract image features at different semantic levels while learning different and subtle features with differences.

8.3.3 *Custom classifications*

For a screening system, high sensitivity and specificity guarantee low misdiagnosis rate and missed diagnosis rate. Different classifier algorithms have various summarizing capabilities for high-level features provided by the bottom feature extractor and consequently greatly affect the prediction performance of the basic learners due to specific datasets and different tasks. Therefore, after attempting rich experiments to explore more suitable classifiers for our work, two classifiers were proposed to provide a basis for a more accurate classification.

For the first system, a classifier ("CFN") was developed via two convolution blocks and several fully connected layers (Fig. 8.4(a)). In the two convolution blocks, 32 and 64 convolution kernels (all 3×3) were used for further feature abstraction and dimension reduction, respectively. The ReLU function was then utilized for nonlinear mapping between hidden layer neurons; a 2×2 maximum pooling layer

Softmax
Dropout layer (0.5)
Dense512-ReLu
Flatten layer
Dropout layer (0.25)
Max pooling layer
32 (3×3) Conv-ReLu
Dropout layer (0.25)
Max pooling layer
64 (3×3) Conv-ReLu

(a) CFN

Softmax
Dropout layer (0.5)
Dense256-LeakyReLu (0.1)
Dropout layer (0.5)
Dense512-LeakyReLu (0.1)
Dropout layer (0.5)
Dense1024-LeakyReLu (0.1)
Dropout layer (0.5)
Dense2048-LeakyReLu (0.1)
Global pooling layer

(b) FCP

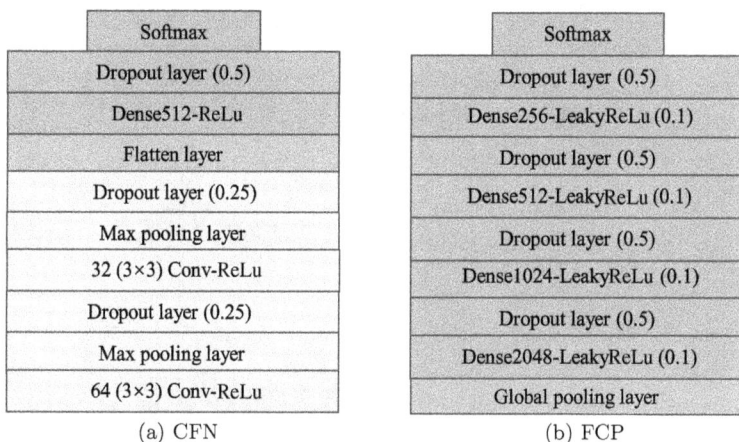

Fig. 8.4. Two custom classifiers. (a) Convolutional layers were used to reduce network parameters further and make training more controllable. The rectified linear unit (ReLU) function was used to alleviate the gradient disappearance problem effectively and make the model converge faster when using the SGD gradient descent method. Hence, CFN was ideal for the simpler binary classification tasks in this study. (b) FC layers were used to reduce the network dimension and complete the implied semantic expression. The leaky ReLU function helped the network attain a strong, robust gradient. Hence, FCP was more suitable for multi-classification tasks.

was used for feature compression. Further, a dropout layer was added to improve the generalization performance of the model. Following layer flattening, the data were transformed into one-dimensional space and further compressed into 512 dimensions using a full connection layer. Finally, the softmax function was used to output the normal and abnormal probability values.

For the latter two systems, a five-layer fully connected perception classifier ('FCP') was designed, shown as in Fig. 8.4(b). The first layer was the global average pooling layer, which could summarize the spatial information from the forward layer, standardize the entire the network structure, prevent overfitting, and reduce the burden of model training. The next four fully connected layers contained 2048, 1024, 512, and 256 hidden neurons. The depths of these layers were very important, such that adding or deleting a single layer could reduce the learning ability of the network, especially with respect to its sensitivity. Leaky ReLU layers and dropout layers ($p = 0.1$) were added after each dense layer. The final layer comprised a softmax layer, which provided corresponding category probabilities based on the characteristics of different tasks.

The two functions of ReLU and leaky ReLU are defined in Eqs. (8.1) and (8.2), respectively.

$$h^{(i)} = \max(w^{(i)(T)}x, 0) = \begin{cases} w^{(i)T}x, & \text{if } w^{(i)T}x > 0 \\ 0, & \text{otherwise,} \end{cases} \qquad (8.1)$$

$$h^{(i)} = \max(w^{(i)(T)}x, 0) = \begin{cases} w^{(i)T}x, & \text{if } w^{(i)T}x > 0 \\ 0.01w^{(i)T}x, & \text{otherwise.} \end{cases} \qquad (8.2)$$

The above formulas show the similarities and differences between the two functions. The latter function may achieve a more robust gradient than the former by sacrificing sparsity, so it is more suitable for the complex multi-classification tasks.

8.3.4 *Class imbalance*

In this study, we used 'class_weights' function in Keras to deal with the class imbalance problem. The parameter of it is set to 'auto', which can provide a weight or bias for each class and helps the models to 'automatically pay more attention' to samples from under-represented class and make the contribution of samples from each class equal to the loss.

8.3.5 *Evaluation metrics*

Nine important scalar measures were used to evaluate the learning algorithms from the perspectives of validity and reliability. Accuracy represents the proportion of fundus images with correct classifications, sensitivity represents the proportion of correctly identified abnormal fundus images (for each type of abnormal image), and specificity represents the proportion of correctly identified normal images.

Other indicators were needed to evaluate the model more objectively because of the class imbalance of aims 2 and 3. Precision represents the ratio of correctly predicted positive samples and is mainly used given a serious category imbalance problem. The Kappa coefficient was used to compare the classification results with randomly assigned values, where a higher Kappa coefficient indicates a more accurate classification. The F1_score was also assessed as the harmonic average of precision and sensitivity. The F_measure constitutes the weighted harmonic average of the F1-score. The receiver operating characteristic curve (ROC) and its area under the ROC curve (AUC) value were used to represent the balance between sensitivity and specificity graphically. Youden's index was used to assess the authenticity of the system. These measures are presented in the following:

$$\text{Accuracy} = \frac{\text{TP} + \text{TN}}{\text{TP} + \text{FP} + \text{TN} + \text{FN}}, \tag{8.3}$$

$$\text{Sensitivity} = \frac{\text{TP}}{\text{TP+FN}}, \tag{8.4}$$

$$\text{Specificity} = \frac{\text{TN}}{\text{TN+FP}}, \tag{8.5}$$

$$\text{F1\_score} = \frac{2\text{TP}}{2\text{TP} + \text{FP} + \text{FN}}, \tag{8.6}$$

$$F_\beta = \frac{\left(1 + \beta^2\right) \times \text{Precision} \times \text{recall}}{\beta^2 \times \text{Precision} + \text{recall}}, \tag{8.7}$$

$$\begin{aligned} \text{Youden's index} &= \text{Sensitivity} + \text{Specificity} - 1 \\ &= \frac{\text{TP} \times \text{TN} - \text{FN} \times \text{FP}}{(\text{TP} + \text{FN}) \times (\text{TN} + \text{FP})}, \end{aligned} \tag{8.8}$$

where the samples can be divided into true positives (TP), false positives (FP), true negatives (TN), and false negatives (FN) in accordance with the combination of the real class and the classifier prediction category.

8.4 Experiments

8.4.1 *Experimental setup*

The project was implemented via Keras and performed on an Intel Xeon E5-2620 CPU and NVIDIA Tesla K40 GPU. The images were split into 70% for training, 10% for verification, and 20% for testing.

Five-fold cross-validation was used to assess the models and ensure that each patient was in only one subset.

8.4.2   *Experimental design*

In the clinic, any computer-aided medical system must guarantee high sensitivity and specificity. The data in the first task were evenly distributed. Thus, selecting an appropriate pretraining model for the extraction of high-quality features was important. In the latter two multi-classification tasks, class imbalance and feature similarity between different categories were the main challenges. Therefore, two alternative implementation strategies in addition to transfer learning and ensemble learning techniques were considered. The specific schemes are described in the following:

(1) **Two-step classification strategy:** First, binary classification models are used to distinguish between normal images and images with abnormal signs (or symptoms). Achieving a good compromise between sensitivity and specificity is the focus of training at this stage. The four-class classification models are then used to identify abnormal signs or diagnose retinal diseases. The focus of this phase is to identify samples of minority classes in the context of class imbalance.

(2) **One-step strategy:** Five-class classification models are trained directly on the sign dataset that includes normal fundus images or on the disease dataset that includes normal fundus images. All the key points in the above strategy are also considered in this strategy.

For more information about tasks under the two strategies, see Table 8.3.

8.4.3   *Screening system*

During the development of the screening system (T1), based on the D1 dataset, the step learning method was used for the learning rate. The rate was initially 2e-5 and decreased to 2e-10 with a constant step size of 0.5. RMSprop was used as an optimizer during the training, and SGD was used during the fine-tuning phase. By means of feature reuse and bypass settings, the DenseNet201 network substantially reduced the number of network parameters

Table 8.3. Task details under different strategies.

Dataset	Data size	Task
D1	8777 images	T1: screening for fundus abnormalities
D2	4541 images	T2: identification of the presence or absence of abnormal signs
D3	3822 images	T3: identification of the four fundus abnormal sign areas
D4	4541 images	T4: identification including normal fundus and four abnormal sign areas
D5	3429 images	T5: diagnose of the presence or absence of abnormal symptoms
D6	2710 images	T6: diagnose of the four fundus diseases
D7	3429 images	T7: diagnose including normal fundus and four abnormal diseases

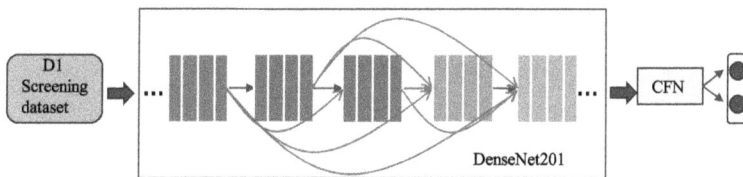

Fig. 8.5. The method of the fundus screening system.

and mitigated gradient loss and model degradation issues, thereby demonstrating better predictive power compared with Inception series models that exhibited wider network structures. Therefore, after extensive experimental comparison, the DenseNet201 pretraining model was adopted as the internal feature extractor of the system, and CFN was used as its classifier. The screening system is shown in Fig. 8.5.

8.4.4 *Sign identification system*

The sign identification task aims to complete the classification of healthy retinas and four abnormal retinal sign areas: optic disc lesion, retinopathy, macular lesion, and vitreous lesion. The step learning method was used for this task. Network training was interrupted after 10 complete passes if the loss of the validation set was no longer reduced.

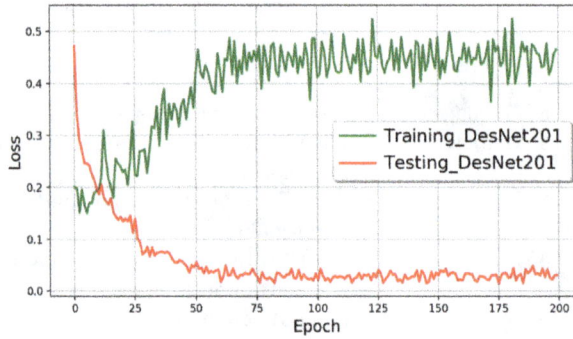

(a) Loss curves

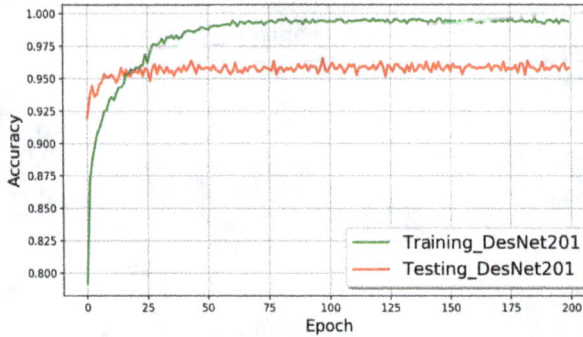

(b) Accuracy curves

Fig. 8.6.   The performance of the screening system.

8.4.4.1   *Two-step classification strategy*

In the experiment, SGD was adopted as an optimizer with a basic learning rate of 0.01 and a momentum of 0.9. It was used to train two binary classification models and three four-class classification models. The D2 dataset was used in the binary classification stage (T2), with feature extractors comprising an InceptionV3 pretraining model and an IncepResnetV2 pretraining model, and their classifiers all used the same CFN classifier. An average method was used to build the binary classification model ('Ensemble2').

In the following four-class classification stage (T3), an Xception pretraining model was used as the third feature extractor in addition to the above two pretraining models, and the feature extractors all used the same FCP classification. Three basic learners were trained using the D3 dataset and then combined into a four-class ensemble model ('Ensemble3').

8.4.4.2 *One-step classification strategy*

The one-step strategy experiment (T4) comprised a five-class classification task based on the D4 dataset. An Adam optimizer was adopted to train the alternative basic learners with an initial learning rate of 2e-4 (beta 1:0.9, beta 2:0.999). After extensive comparison experiments, three Inception models were selected as the basic learners; these consisted of the above three Inception pretraining models used as feature extractors and three FCNs used for inner classifications.

8.4.5 *Disease diagnosis system*

Regarding the disease diagnosis system, classification imbalance was also pronounced, particularly for RT, which constituted only 2% of the disease dataset and tended to be frequently identified as RD (Table 8.8). Therefore, two alternative implementation strategies were also considered.

8.4.5.1 *Two-step classification strategy*

In the binary class stage, based on the D5 dataset, three new learners were trained independently. These learners comprised the Xception learner, InceptionResNetV2 learner, Inceptionv3 learner, and their respective CFNs. $lr = 2e - 5$ was used as the initial value, and this value was reduced by a factor of 0.5 per 10 epochs. RMSprop optimizer and SGD optimizer ($lr = 0.001$) were used during training and fine-tuning, respectively. A weighted stacking method was used to build the ensemble model ('Ensemble5').

In the four-class classification stage, another set of Inception learners was independently trained, and their classifiers were replaced with three new FCPs. The SGD optimizer with a basic learning rate of 0.01 and a momentum of 0.9 was used during the training. Finally, the three basic learners were integrated ('Ensemble6') by averaging their softmax scores due to their different output magnitudes. Based on the D6 dataset, Ensemble6 achieved a good average accuracy of 96.13%.

8.4.5.2 *One-step classification strategy*

In the five-class classification experiment, the above three pretraining feature extractors and their corresponding FCPs were combined to build the ensemble model ('Ensemble7'). The new five-class basic learners were trained based on the D7 dataset. The SGD optimizer was used during the training phase, and the RMSprop optimizer was used during the fine-tuning phase.

8.4.6 *Result*

8.4.6.1 *Screening system*

Table 8.4 shows that the fundus screening system performed well. Accuracy was 97.33%, sensitivity was 96.04%, and specificity was 93.83% on the ZS dataset. Details of training and classification on these images are shown in Fig. 8.7.

8.4.6.2 *Sign identification system*

(1) **Two-step classification strategy:** Table 8.5 shows that, for Ensemble2, the average accuracy was 97.14%, sensitivity was 97.75%, and specificity was 94.04%. Table 8.6 shows that for Ensemble3, average accuracy was 93.92%; its precision values were 88% for optic papillary alteration, 96% for retinopathy, 88% for macular lesion, and 67% for vitreous lesion. The main reason for the 67% precision for vitreous lesion may be that only 98 images included vitreous lesions, which comprised 2.1% of the training dataset.

(2) **One-step classification strategy:** The average accuracy of the final ensemble (Ensemble4) using the one-step strategy was 91.62%; sensitivity and specificity were 92.28% and 96.3%, respectively. These values did not exceed the performance of Ensemble3 in the four-category strategy.

8.4.6.3 *Disease diagnosis system*

(1) **Two-step classification strategy:** Table 8.7 shows that Ensemble5 achieved an average accuracy of 98.25%, a sensitivity of 99.26%, and a specificity of 94.44%. Based on the D6 dataset, Ensemble6 achieved a good average accuracy of 96.13%. Table 8.8 shows

Table 8.4. Performances of the screening system.

Model	Source	Classifier	Image	ACC	SEN	SPE	PREC	AUC	kappa	F1_s	F_m	YI
BL1	ZS	CFN	2603	94.66	93.30	95.45	94.16	94.37	88.53	94.26	94.20	88.75
System	ZS	CFN	2603	96.04	93.83	97.33	95.89	95.58	91.46	96.04	95.82	91.16
	SC	CFN	421	93.11	90.24	95.83	93.26	93.04	86.20	93.10	93.19	86.08
	MY	CFN	1343	94.48	89.82	97.18	94.12	93.50	87.98	94.46	94.32	87.00

Notes: ACC: accuracy, SEN: sensitivity, SPE: specificity, PRE: precision, F1_s: F1_score, F_m: F_meature, YI: Youden's index. BL1 is a DensNet169 network used as baseline in T1 task.

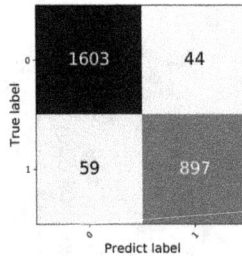

(a) CM1

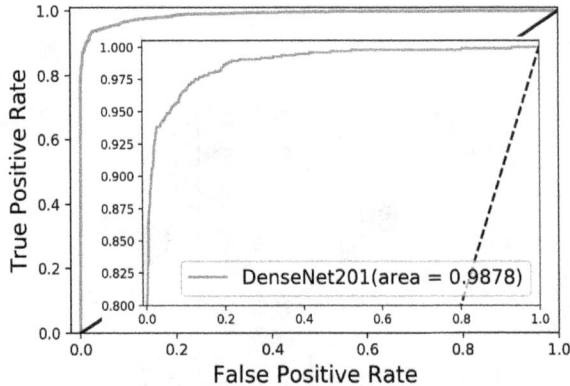

(b) ROC curve

Fig. 8.7. The screening system. (a) CM1: The confusion matrix of the system was DensNet201. (b) The ROC curve was drawn with sensitivity as the ordinate and (1-specificity) as the abscissa. The larger the area under the curve, the higher the diagnostic accuracy, and vice versa. On the ROC curve, the point closest to the upper left of the graph was the critical value with higher sensitivity and specificity. The small figure of (a) is a magnification of the curve in the upper left corner for clarity, and the same is true for Figs. 8.10 and 8.14.

that the precision rates of RD, RT, DR, and myopia were 98%, 75%, 94%, and 89%, respectively; the main reason for the low precision of RT was mainly related to its minority class. The confusion matrix in Fig. 8.13(c) demonstrates that of the six RT images misidentified by Ensemble6, three and three were misclassified as RD and myopia, respectively. The main reasons are speculated to include the limited number of training images of RT, the common clinical progression from RT to RD, and the role of myopia as a risk factor for RT during symptomatic posterior vitreous detachment.

Table 8.5.   Comparison of the performance of identification models via the two strategies.

Task	Model	Classifier	ACC	SEN	SPE	PREC	Recall	Kappa	F1_score	F_meature	YI
BL2	DesNet169	CFN	93.83	95.77	84.10	93.83	89.93	78.22	93.89	93.94	79.87
T2											
D2	InResv2	CFN	96.48	97.23	92.72	96.60	94.97	87.61	96.52	96.57	89.94
	Incepv3	CFN	96.04	96.96	91.39	96.17	94.17	86.07	96.08	92.39	88.35
	Ens2	CFN	**97.14**	**97.75**	**94.04**	**97.22**	**95.90**	**89.89**	**97.17**	**97.20**	**91.79**
BL3	DesNet169	CFN	90.48	/	/	89.72	62.72	69.25	89.93	89.76	/
T3											
D3	InResv2	FCP	92.87	/	/	92.47	72.92	77.64	92.58	92.50	/
	Incepv3	FCP	90.75	/	/	90.08	66.05	70.50	90.23	89.92	/
	Xcep	FCP	92.07	/	/	91.43	68.47	75.26	91.64	91.48	/
	Ens3	FCP	**93.92**	/	/	**93.53**	**74.18**	**80.81**	**93.92**	**93.52**	/
	SP	FCP	89.06	/	/	90.27	89.06	81.51	86.27	89.41	/
	MY	FCP	90.19	/	/	89.14	90.19	79.82	89.44	89.20	/
BL4	DesNet169	FCP	88.76	83.44	95.51	88.76	71.64	77.46	88.49	88.46	78.95
T4											
D4	InResv2	FCP	91.51	96.43	93.38	91.61	76.00	83.21	91.33	91.42	89.81
	Incepv3	FCP	90.41	96.57	91.39	90.37	74.97	80.98	90.26	90.29	87.96
	Xcep	FCP	90.74	97.10	86.09	90.57	75.02	81.31	90.45	90.74	83.19
	Ens4	FCP	91.62	96.83	92.72	91.57	74.23	83.18	91.31	91.37	89.54

Notes: InResv2: InceptionResnetv2, Incepv3: Inceptionv3, Xcep: Xception, Ens3: Ensemble3, Ens4: Ensemble4. BL2–BL4 are the three DensNet169 networks used as baselines in T2–T4 tasks.

(a) Loss curves

(b) Accuracy curves

(c) CM2

(d) ROC curves

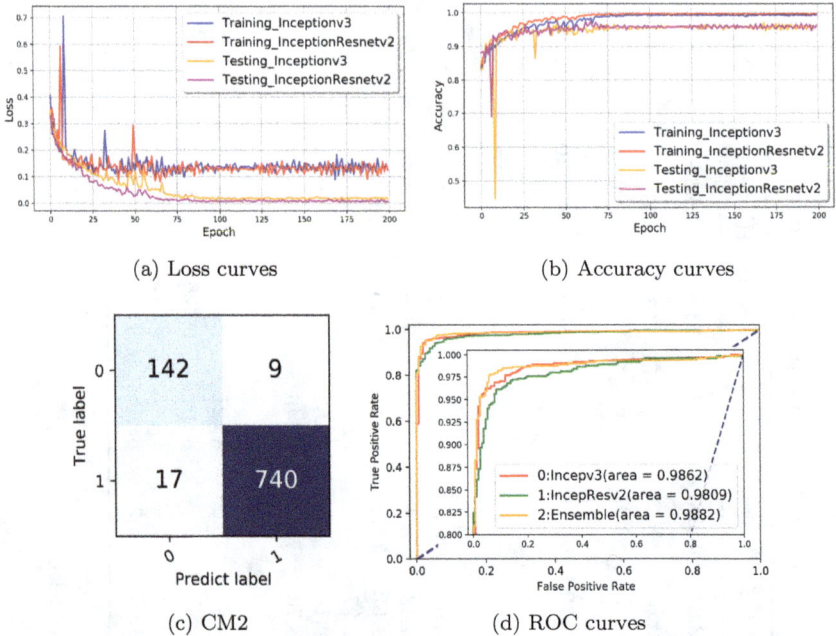

Fig. 8.8.   The performance on binary classification task by CM2. (c) 0: normal and 1: abnormal. (a) and (b) show the loss curves and accuracy curves of components during training and testing in the binary classification task.

Table 8.6.   Class distribution and classifications report of the identification system.

Class	Training	Testing	Total	Class	Precision	Recall	F1_score	Support
0	568	151	719	1	88	82	85	91
1	404	91	495	2	96	99	97	609
2	2464	609	3073	3	88	74	80	38
3	118	38	156	4	67	42	52	19
4	79	19	98	Micro avg	94	94	94	757

Notes: 0: normal, 1: optic disc lesion, 2: retinopathy, 3: macular lesions, 4: vitreous lesion.

(2) One-step classification strategy: Table 8.7 shows that the prediction accuracy of Ensemble7 was 95.33%, sensitivity was 98.89%, and specificity was 97.92%; these values did not exceed the performance of Ensemble6 in the four-category strategy.

Table 8.7. The comparison of the performance of the diagnostic models under the two strategies (in bold).

Task	Model	Classifier	ACC	SEN	SPE	PREC	Recall	Kappa	F1_score	F_meature	YI
BI5	DesNet169	CFN	94.89	95.20	93.75	91.06	94.47	85.25	94.99	95.13	88.95
T5											
D5	InResv2	CFN	97.81	98.71	94.44	96.81	96.57	93.39	96.70	96.76	93.15
	Incepv3	CFN	97.38	98.89	91.67	96.73	95.27	91.97	95.98	96.42	90.56
	Xcep	CFN	97.67	98.52	94.44	96.48	96.48	92.97	96.48	96.48	92.97
	Ens5	CFN	**98.25**	**99.26**	**94.44**	**97.83**	**96.51**	**94.67**	**97.33**	**98.24**	**93.70**
BI6	DesNet169	FCP	92.98	/	/	92.65	74.15	83.79	92.51	92.49	/
T6											
D6	InResv2	FCP	95.94	/	/	95.82	81.90	92.18	95.71	95.71	/
	Incepv3	FCP	95.57	/	/	95.52	85.10	91.10	95.54	95.52	/
	Xcep	FCP	95.38	/	/	95.26	83.38	90.48	95.26	95.24	/
	Ens6	FCP	**96.13**	/	/	**96.03**	**84.61**	**92.39**	**96.01**	**96.00**	/
	SP	FCP	93.17	/	/	90.77	93.17	77.93	91.75	91.11	/
	MY	FCP	93.69	/	/	94.12	93.68	83.03	92.98	93.17	/
BI7	DesNet169	FCP	89.36	97.8	91.67	68.06	70.48	82.52	88.65	68.51	89.47
T7											
D7	InResv2	FCP	92.13	97.60	97.92	90.96	74.46	86.22	91.40	91.11	95.52
	Incepv3	FCP	94.31	99.01	95.83	93.79	78.07	88.92	93.95	93.81	92.13
	Xcep	FCP	95.19	98.89	95.14	95.04	82.35	88.60	95.00	94.98	94.03
	Ens7	FCP	95.34	98.89	97.22	95.05	81.05	89.76	95.05	95.00	96.12

Notes: Ens5: Ensemble5, Ens6: Ensemble6, Ens7: Ensemble7. BL5–BL7 are the three DensNet169 networks used as baselines in T5–T7 tasks.

(a) Loss curves

(b) Accuracy curves

(c) CM3

(d) ROC curves

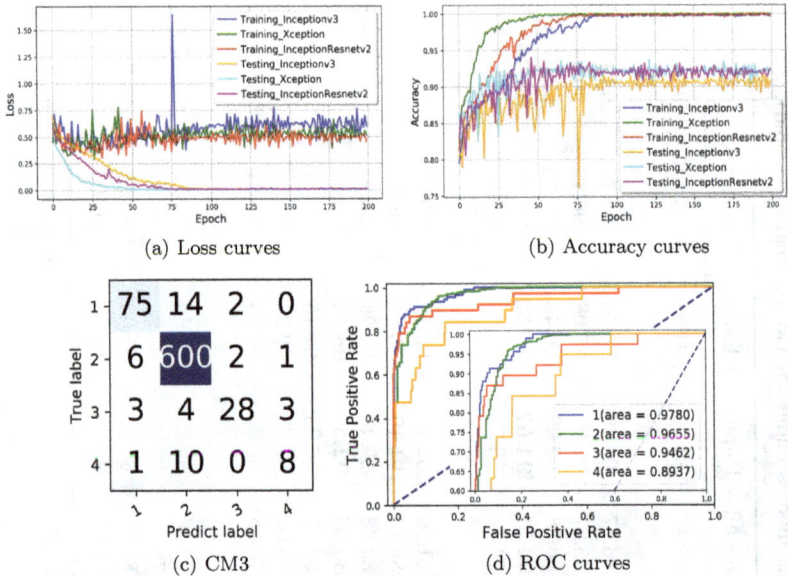

Fig. 8.9.   The performance on four-class classification task by CM3. (c) 0: normal, 1: optic disc lesion, 2: retinopathy, 3: macular lesion, and 4: vitreous lesion. (a) and (b) show the loss curves and accuracy curves of components during training and testing in the four-category task.

Table 8.8.   Class distribution and classifications report of the diagnose system.

Class	Training	Testing	Total	Class	Precision	Recall	F1_score	Support
Normal	575	144	719	RD	98	98	98	390
RD	1526	390	1916	RT	75	50	60	12
RT	58	12	70	DR	94	98	96	81
DR	309	81	390	Myopia	89	93	91	59
Myopia	275	59	334	Avg	96	96	96	542

8.4.7   *Comparative experiments*

For objectivity, a set of benchmark experiments were carried out using the DenseNet169 pretraining model as the feature extractor that was connected to the corresponding task classifier. DenseNet169 was selected because it has relatively low parameters compared with other models, and the architecture handles the vanish gradient problem well. For convenience, these baseline experiments were named BL1–BL7 to correspond to Tasks T1–T7, respectively. The results demonstrate that the feature extractors of the system and the two-step strategy were more effective in our study. Tables 8.4, 8.5, and 8.7 provide further details.

8.4.8 Generalization performance

Two additional datasets were collected during manuscript preparation and used to evaluate the generalization performance of the DeepUWF-Plus method. The first additional dataset was from the Department of Ophthalmology of Sichuan Provincial People's Hospital (SC), and the second dataset was from the Department of Ophthalmology of Mianyang Central Hospital (MY). Table 8.2 depicts the specific data distributions. Table 8.4 shows that the accuracy, sensitivity, and specificity of the screening system were 93.11%, 90.24%, and 95.83% for SC, respectively, and 94.48%, 89.82%, and 97.18% for MY, respectively. Table 8.5 shows that the accuracy and average precision of the identification system were 89.06% and 89.14% for the SC dataset, respectively, and 90.19% and 89.14% for the MY dataset, respectively. Table 8.7 shows that the accuracy and average precision of the diagnosis system were 93.17% and 90.77% for the SC dataset, respectively, and 93.69% and 94.12% for the MY dataset, respectively.

8.5 Discussion

8.5.1 Comparison of the two strategies

During the development of the sign identification system, the two-step strategy achieved a better local optimal solution and exhibited a better average accuracy regarding the sign lesions (Fig. 8.10, 8.12, and 8.13). Implementation of Ensemble3 using the two-step strategy improved the recognition accuracies of two types of signs: optic papillary alteration and retinopathy. For the two-step strategy, a positive sample presumed missed in the binary class stage could be correctly identified in the subsequent stage of sign four-class classification. If not correctly identified, it was only a shift between related sign types

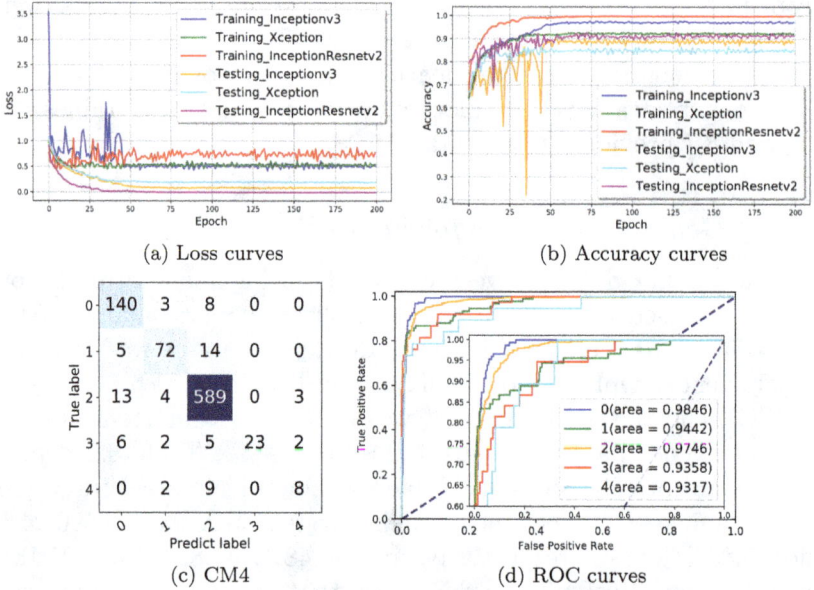

(a) Loss curves

(b) Accuracy curves

(c) CM4

(d) ROC curves

Fig. 8.10. The performance on five-class classification task by CM3. (c) 0: normal, 1: optic disc lesion, 2: retinopathy, 3: macular lesion, and 4: vitreous lesion. (a) and (b) show the loss curves and accuracy curves of components during training and testing in the five-category task.

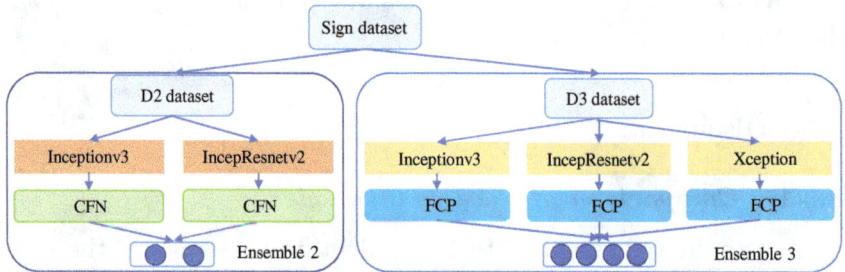

Fig. 8.11. The method of the identification system.

in positive samples, which did not affect sensitivity, fundamentally reducing the rate of missed diagnosis in positive samples. Moreover, the DensNet169 network in the benchmark experiment also showed that its prediction performance under the two-stage strategy was better than that under the one-step strategy. Finally, the sign identification system was implemented, as shown in Fig. 8.11.

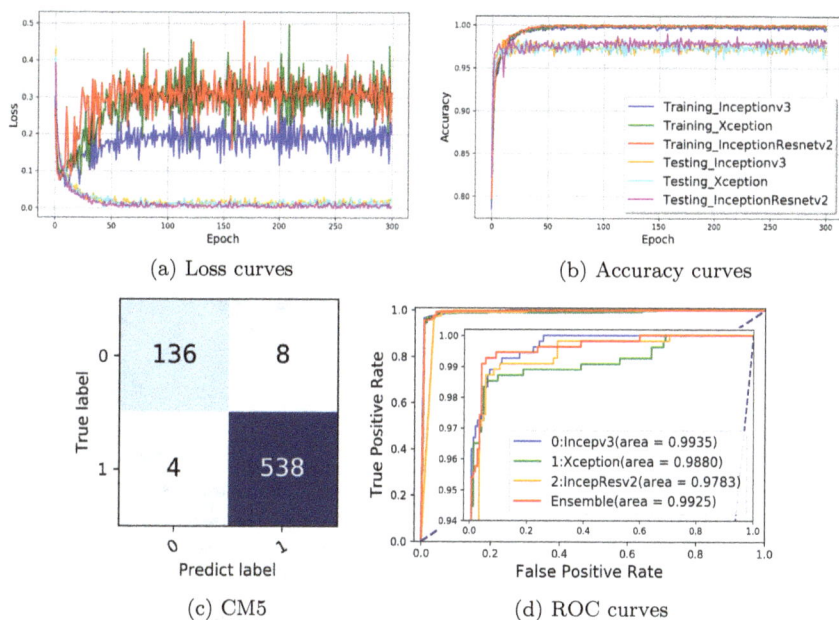

(a) Loss curves   (b) Accuracy curves

(c) CM5   (d) ROC curves

Fig. 8.12. The performance on binary classification task by CM5. (c) 0: normal, 1: abnormal. (a) and (b) show the loss curves and accuracy curves of components during training and testing in this task.

During the development of the disease diagnosis system, Fig. 8.14 revealed intuitively that the strategy of the four-class classification was optimal. The two-step strategy can perform a secondary check on the prediction of the positive disease sample. Although several positive samples were misdiagnosed in the previous binary classification, they may be corrected in the following four-class classification stage. Regardless of whether these positive samples were misdiagnosed as other fundus eye diseases, the risk of misdiagnosis was greatly reduced. Moreover, DensNet169, the baseline network in the system, also showed a better prediction performance under the two-stage strategy than under the one-step strategy. Finally, the disease diagnostic system was implemented, as shown in Fig. 8.15.

8.5.2 Model performance

Tertiary hospitals often receive patients with various refractory retinal diseases from different locations nationwide, and their fundus

(a) Loss curves

(b) Accuracy curves

(c) CM6

(d) ROC curves

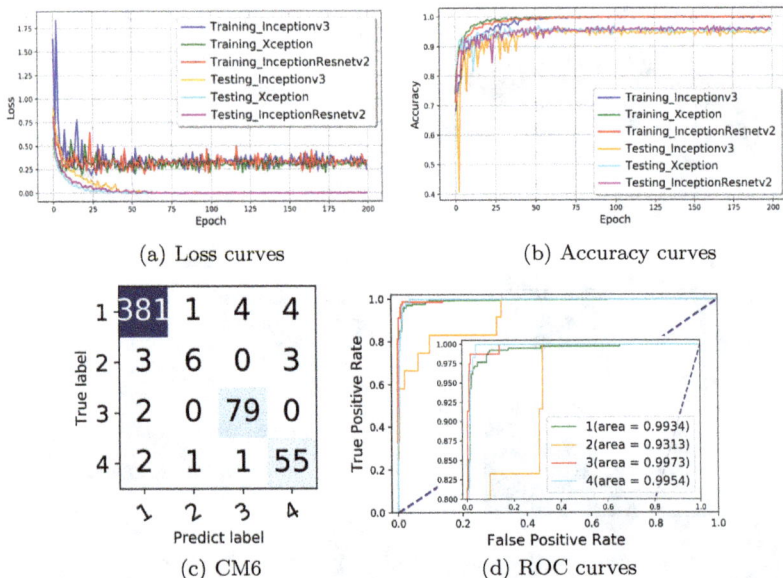

Fig. 8.13.   The performance on four-class classification task by CM6. (c) 0: normal, 1: optic disc lesion, 2: retinopathy, 3: macular lesion, and 4: vitreous lesion.

images are complex. However, the scale of collected data is limited, and these factors create additional challenges regarding classification tasks. Our research results show that the DeepUWF-Plus model, based on the two-step classification strategy, has better prediction performance than the one-step classification strategy. Nevertheless, DL models may detect several subtle abnormalities that are not identified by clinicians, which can affect model performance. Moreover, dataset heterogeneity among hospitals, differences in acquisition equipment, and differences in imaging parameters are important factors in a model's generalization performance. Additional data from different hospitals and joint assessment of data among multiple hospitals are needed to extract various representative medical features that can improve the performance of each hospital's model.

8.5.3 *Medical implication*

This system provides a basis for establishing a deep fundus screening service. First, the UWF images used in this study exhibit a

(a) Loss curves

(b) Accuracy curves

(c) CM7

(d) ROC curves

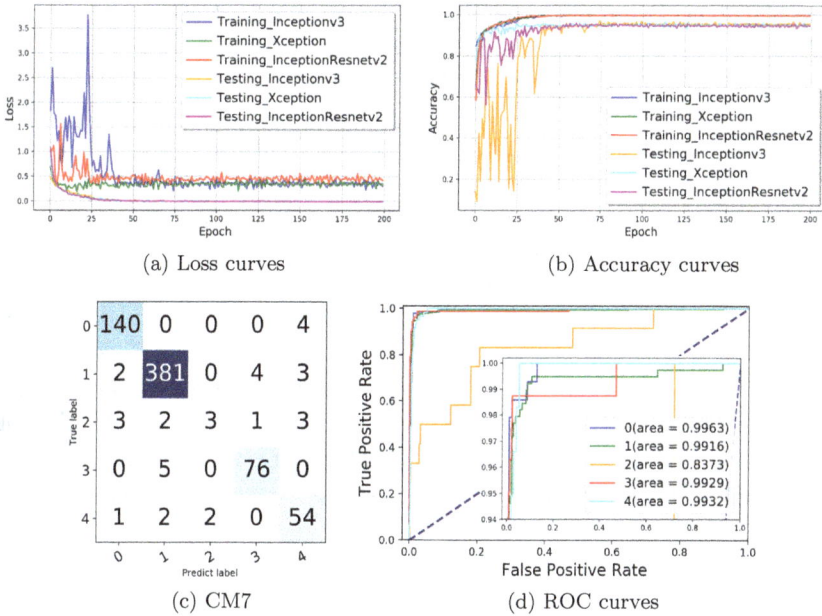

Fig. 8.14. The disease diagnostic system. (c) 0: normal, 1: RD, 2: RT, 3: DR, and 4: myopia. (a) and (b) show the loss curves and accuracy curves of each learner in training and testing in the five-class classification task. (d) reflects those of Ensemble7 in the five-category task.

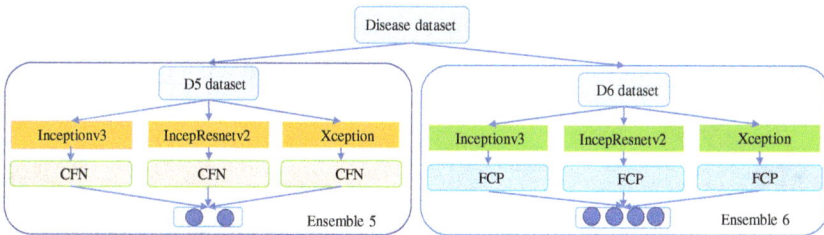

Fig. 8.15. The method of the disease diagnostic system.

large number of pathological fundus signs of common retinal diseases in China. This diversity of retinal information helps heterogeneous populations participate more easily in screening efforts for fundus abnormalities and improves the accessibility of eye care services in rural or remote areas.

Second, the performance of retinal disease screening is an extremely urgent task. DR patients are 25-fold more likely to develop blindness. Pathological myopia is an important risk factor for serious eye conditions, which considerably increases the likelihood of RT by 21-fold. RT always leads to RD, but their treatment and prevention are cost-effective compared with other retinal diseases, regardless of treatment modality (Chang and Smiddy, 2014). A retinal disease diagnosis subsystem helps inspectors assess the risk of disease in the general public and enhances the feasibility of evaluation.

Fundus sign screening provides important insights into the early diagnosis and treatment of most retinal diseases and several systemic diseases. For example, the optic nerve is an extension of the brain, and DR is a chronic complication of diabetes. The detection of abnormal signs in clinical examinations is more reliable, comprehensive, and in depth compared with diagnosis based on patient-reported symptoms.

8.5.4 *Research limitations*

We acknowledge that the gradient disappearance problem in DL makes the model favor the local optimal solution. In the context of a limited dataset, class imbalance hinders the equal representation of data types, which makes learning prefer majority classes and exhibit poor generalization. Furthermore, the labeling task was performed based on the clinical experience of the ophthalmologists involved. Thus, the algorithm may behave differently given subtle signs or symptoms in the images used that most clinicians cannot recognize.

8.5.5 *Future work*

In the follow-up work, large-scale data acquisition may alleviate these problems and improve system performance. Other imaging modalities may also need to be combined for further exploration of the staging and typing of these diseases as well as accurate examination and diagnosis because many retinal diseases have different treatment options at different stages.

8.6 DeepUWF: An AI System for Multiple Fundus Diseases Diagnosis

Timely detection and accurate diagnosis of fundus lesions are essential to protect the eye health. Based on the proposed model, DeepUWF, an intelligent screening system for abnormal signs of fundus and an intelligent diagnosis system for multiple diseases, was developed in our work. The DeepUWF adopts B/S architecture. The doctors log into the system through the browser and upload ultrawide-angle fundus images. The cloud server receives and stores the corresponding image information, and then uses the proposed deep neural networks to analyze and predict the diagnosis of the image. The prediction results are submitted to the clinician for review and correction. The final diagnosis report is written into the corresponding database and returned to the user interface in PDF format. The framework of the DeepUWF is shown in Fig. 5.16.

At present, the DeepUWF has been put into the clinical trial at Sichuan Provincial People's Hospital. The system operation interface is shown in Fig. 8.16. The clinical test shows that the recognition rate of the system in the left and right eyes is as high as 97.23%, the

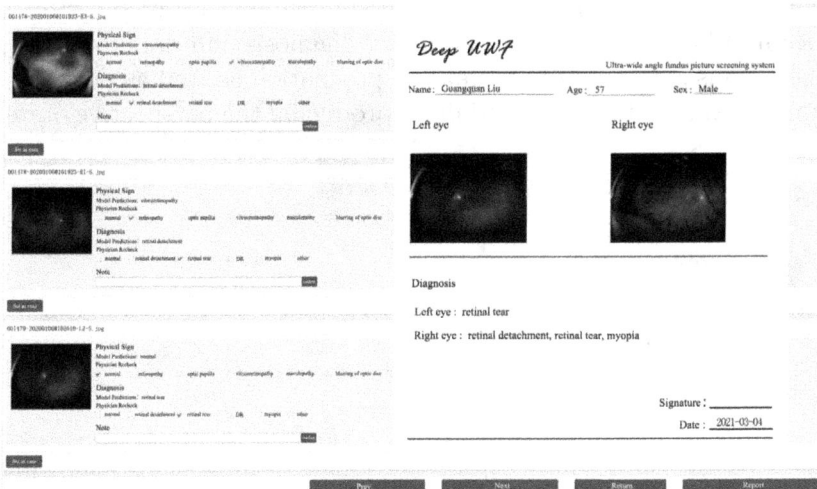

Fig. 8.16. The system operation interface of DeepUWF.

accuracy rate in the detection of pathological signs is about 85.23%, and the accuracy rate in the diagnosis of ocular fundus diseases is about 92.44%.

8.7 Conclusion

In this study, a UWF imaging medical dataset was established, and two customized multi-layer perceptions were designed as classifiers and combined with advanced CNNs via transfer learning to form multiple learners. An auxiliary fundus screening system (DeepUWF-Plus), which consists of three modules, namely, an abnormal fundus screening subsystem, an abnormal sign identification subsystem, and a disease diagnosis subsystem, was also developed. Data augmentation technology was applied to improve data diversity and system generalization.

The effects of two-step and one-step classification strategies on the predictive performance of recognition and diagnosis models were experimentally analyzed to meet the dual challenges of unbalanced classification and between-class similarity. The performances of the models were evaluated with respect to effectiveness and reliability. The experimental results showed that the two-stage classification strategy helped improve the predictive abilities of the models. DeepUWF-Plus may enable auxiliary diagnosis and data analysis in the fundus screening of the general population as well as outpatient fundus examinations by partially reproducing the perspective of retinal experts.

Bibliography

Abadi, M., Agarwal, A., Barham, P., Brevdo, E., Chen, Z., Citro, C., Corrado, G. S., Davis, A., Dean, J., Devin, M., *et al.* (2016). Tensorflow: Large-scale machine learning on heterogeneous distributed systems, *arXiv preprint arXiv:1603.04467*.

Abelson, S., Collord, G., and Ng, S. (2018). Prediction of acute myeloid leukaemia risk in healthy individuals, *Nature* **559**, 400–404.

Abràmoff, M. D., Garvin, M. K., and Sonka, M. (2010). Retinal imaging and image analysis, *IEEE Reviews in Biomedical Engineering* **3**, 169–208.

Abràmoff, M. D., Lavin, P. T., Birch, M., Shah, N., and Folk, J. C. (2018). Pivotal trial of an autonomous ai-based diagnostic system for detection of diabetic retinopathy in primary care offices, *Npj Digital Medicine* **1**(1), 1–8.

Abràmoff, M. D., Lou, Y., Erginay, A., Clarida, W., Amelon, R., Folk, J. C., and Niemeijer, M. (2016). Improved automated detection of diabetic retinopathy on a publicly available dataset through integration of deep learning, *Investigative Ophthalmology & Visual Science* **57**(13), 5200–5206.

Adarsh, P. and Jeyakumari, D. (2013). Multiclass svm-based automated diagnosis of diabetic retinopathy, in *2013 International Conference on Communication and Signal Processing*, pp. 206–210, doi: 10.1109/iccsp.2013.6577044.

Ahlers, C., Simader, C., Geitzenauer, W., Stock, G., Stetson, P., Dastmalchi, S., and Schmidt-Erfurth, U. (2008). Automatic segmentation in three-dimensional analysis of fibrovascular pigmentepithelial detachment using high-definition optical coherence tomography, *British Journal of Ophthalmology* **92**(2), 197–203.

Akram, M. U., Khalid, S., Tariq, A., Khan, S. A., and Azam, F. (2014). Detection and classification of retinal lesions for grading of diabetic retinopathy, *Computers in Biology and Medicine* **45**, 161–171.

Al-Diri, B., Hunter, A., Steel, D., Habib, M., Hudaib, T., and Berry, S. (2008). Review – a reference data set for retinal vessel profiles, in *2008 30th Annual International Conference of the IEEE Engineering in Medicine and Biology Society*, pp. 2262–2265. doi: 10.1109/IEMBS.2008.4649647.

Albarqouni, S., Baur, C., Achilles, F., Belagiannis, V., Demirci, S., and Navab, N. (2016). Aggnet: Deep learning from crowds for mitosis detection in breast cancer histology images, *IEEE Transactions on Medical Imaging* **35**(5), 1313–1321.

Anthimopoulos, M., Christodoulidis, S., Ebner, L., Christe, A., and Mougiakakou, S. (2016). Lung pattern classification for interstitial lung diseases using a deep convolutional neural network, *IEEE Transactions on Medical Imaging* **35**(5), 1207–1216.

Asaoka, R., Murata, H., Iwase, A., and Araie, M. (2016). Detecting preperimetric glaucoma with standard automated perimetry using a deep learning classifier, *Ophthalmology* **123**(9), 1974–1980. doi: https://doi.org/10.1016/j.ophtha.2016.05.029.

Aslam, T., Fleck, B., Patton, N., Trucco, M., and Azegrouz, H. (2009). Digital image analysis of plus disease in retinopathy of prematurity, *Acta Ophthalmologica* **87**(4), 368–377.

Ataer-Cansizoglu, E., Bolon-Canedo, V., Campbell, J. P., Bozkurt, A., Erdogmus, D., Kalpathy-Cramer, J., Patel, S., Jonas, K., Chan, R. P., Ostmo, S., *et al.* (2015). Computer-based image analysis for plus disease diagnosis in retinopathy of prematurity: Performance of the "i-rop" system and image features associated with expert diagnosis, *Translational Vision Science Technology* **4**(6), 5.

Aylward, S. R. and Bullitt, E. (2002). Initialization, noise, singularities, and scale in height ridge traversal for tubular object centerline extraction, *IEEE Transactions on Medical Imaging* **21**(2), 61–75.

Badrinarayanan, V., Kendall, A., and Cipolla, R. (2017). Segnet: A deep convolutional encoder-decoder architecture for image segmentation, *IEEE Transactions on Pattern Analysis and Machine Intelligence* **39**(12), 2481–2495.

Bagheri, N., Wajda, B. N., Calvo, C. M., Durrani, A. K., Friedberg, M. A., and Rapuano, C. J. (2017). *The Wills Eye Manual: Office and Emergency Room Diagnosis and Treatment of Eye Disease*. Philadelphia: Wolters Kluwer.

Bas, E., Ataer-Cansizoglu, E., Erdogmus, D., and Kalpathy-Cramer, J. (2012). Retinal vasculature segmentation using principal spanning forests, in *Biomedical Imaging (ISBI), 2012 9th IEEE International Symposium on*, pp. 1792–1795.

Bengio, Y., Courville, A., and Vincent, P. (2013). Representation learning: A review and new perspectives, *IEEE Transactions on Pattern Analysis and Machine Intelligence* **35**(8), 1798–1828.

Bengio, Y., Lamblin, P., Popovici, D., and Larochelle, H. (2007). Greedy layer-wise training of deep networks, in *Advances in Neural Information Processing Systems*, pp. 153–160.

Benson, J., Carrillo, H., Wigdahl, J., Nemeth, S., Maynard, J., Zamora, G., Barriga, S., Estrada, T., and Soliz, P. (2018). Transfer learning for diabetic retinopathy, International Society for Optics and Photonics, p. 105741Z.

Berwick, M. D. and Hackbarth, A. D. (2012). Eliminating waste in us health care, *Jama* **307**(14), 1513–1516.

Bhatkar, A. P. and Kharat, G. U. (2015). Detection of diabetic retinopathy in retinal images using mlp classifier, in *2015 IEEE International Symposium on Nanoelectronic and Information Systems*, pp. 331–335. doi: 10.1109/iNIS.2015.30.

Bloice, M. D., Stocker, C., and Holzinger, A. (2017). Augmentor: An image augmentation library for machine learning, *arXiv preprint arXiv:1708.04680*.

Bolón-Canedo, V., Ataer-Cansizoglu, E., Erdogmus, D., Kalpathy-Cramer, J., Fontenla-Romero, O., Alonso-Betanzos, A., and Chiang, M. F. (2015). Dealing with inter-expert variability in retinopathy of prematurity: A machine learning approach, *Computer Methods and Programs in Biomedicine* **122**(1), 1–15.

Bonab, H. R. and Can, F. (2016). A theoretical framework on the ideal number of classifiers for online ensembles in data streams, pp. 2053–2056.

Bonab, H. R. and Can, F. (2019). Less is more: A comprehensive framework for the number of components of ensemble classifiers, *IEEE Transactions on Neural Networks and Learning Systems* **30**(9), 2735–2745.

Boureau, Y.-L., Ponce, J., and LeCun, Y. (2010). A theoretical analysis of feature pooling in visual recognition, pp. 111–118.

Bourne, R. R. *et al.* (2013). Causes of vision loss worldwide, 1990–2010: A systematic analysis, *The Lancet Global Health* **1**(6), e339–e349.

Bradski, G. (2000). The opencv library, *Dr. Dobb's Journal: Software Tools for the Professional Programmer* **25**(11), 120–123.

Brown, J. M., Campbell, J. P., Beers, A., Chang, K., Ostmo, S., Chan, R. V. P., Dy, J., Erdogmus, D., Ioannidis, S., Kalpathy-Cramer, J., Chiang, M. F., for the Imaging, and in Retinopathy of Prematurity (i ROP) Research Consortium, I. (2018). Automated diagnosis of plus disease in retinopathy of prematurity using deep convolutional neural networks, *JAMA Ophthalmology* **136**(7), 803–810. doi: 10.1001/jamaophthalmol.2018.1934.

Burlina, P., Pacheco, K. D., Joshi, N., Freund, D. E., and Bressler, N. M. (2017). Comparing humans and deep learning performance for grading amd: A study in using universal deep features and transfer learning for automated amd analysis, *Computers in Biology and Medicine* **82**, 80–86, doi: https://doi.org/10.1016/j.compbiomed.2017.01.018.

Campbell, J. P., Kalpathy-Cramer, J., Erdogmus, D., Tian, P., Kedarisetti, D., Moleta, C., Reynolds, J. D., Hutcheson, K., Shapiro, M. J., Repka, M. X., *et al.* (2016). Plus disease in retinopathy of prematurity: A continuous spectrum of vascular abnormality as a basis of diagnostic variability, *Ophthalmology* **123**(11), 2338–2344.

Carneiro, G., Nascimento, J., and Bradley, A. P. (2017). Automated analysis of unregistered multi-view mammograms with deep learning, *IEEE Transactions on Medical Imaging* **36**(11), 2355–2365.

Chandore, V. and Asati, S. (2017). Automatic detection of diabetic retinopathy using deep convolutional neural network, *International Journal of Advance Research, Ideas and Innovations in Technology* **3**, 633–641.

Chang, J. S. and Smiddy, W. E. (2014). Cost-effectiveness of retinal detachment repair, *Ophthalmology* **121**(4), 946–951. doi: https://doi.org/10.1016/j.ophtha.2013.11.003.

Chen, D. and Davies, M. E. (2020). Deep decomposition learning for inverse imaging problems, in *Proceedings of the European Conference on Computer Vision (ECCV)*, pp. 510–526.

Chen, J. and Smith, L. E. (2007). Retinopathy of prematurity, *Angiogenesis* **10**(2), 133–140.

Chen, L.-C., Papandreou, G., Kokkinos, I., Murphy, K., and Yuille, A. L. (2017). Deeplab: Semantic image segmentation with deep convolutional nets, atrous convolution, and fully connected crfs, *IEEE Transactions on Pattern Analysis and Machine Intelligence* **40**(4), 834–848.

Chen, L.-C., Zhu, Y., Papandreou, G., Schroff, F., and Adam, H. (2018). Encoder-decoder with atrous separable convolution for semantic image segmentation, *arXiv preprint arXiv:1802.02611*.

Chen, Q., Leng, T., Zheng, L., Kutzscher, L., Ma, J., de Sisternes, L., and Rubin, D. L. (2013). Automated drusen segmentation and quantification in sd-oct images, *Medical Image Analysis* **17**(8), 1058–1072.

Chen, T., Li, M., Li, Y., Lin, M., Wang, N., Wang, M., Xiao, T., Xu, B., Zhang, C., and Zhang, Z. (2015). Mxnet: A flexible and efficient machine learning library for heterogeneous distributed systems, *arXiv preprint arXiv:1512.01274*.

Chen, X., Niemeijer, M., Zhang, L., Lee, K., Abràmoff, M. D., and Sonka, M. (2012). Three-dimensional segmentation of fluid-associated abnormalities in retinal oct: Probability constrained graph-search-graph-cut, *IEEE Transactions on Medical Imaging* **31**(8), 1521–1531.

Chiang, M. F., Jiang, L., Gelman, R., Du, Y. E., and Flynn, J. T. (2007). Inter-expert agreement of plus disease diagnosis in retinopathy of prematurity, *Archives of Ophthalmology* **125**(7), 875–880.

Chiu, S. J., Allingham, M. J., Mettu, P. S., Cousins, S. W., Izatt, J. A., and Farsiu, S. (2015). Kernel regression based segmentation of optical coherence tomography images with diabetic macular edema, *Biomedical Optics Express* **6**(4), 1172–1194.

Chiu, S. J., Li, X. T., Nicholas, P., Toth, C. A., Izatt, J. A., and Farsiu, S. (2010). Automatic segmentation of seven retinal layers in sdoct images congruent with expert manual segmentation, *Optics Express* **18**(18), 19413–19428.

Choi, J. Y., Yoo, T. K., Seo, J. G., Kwak, J., Um, T. T., and Rim, T. H. (2017). Multi-categorical deep learning neural network to classify retinal images: A pilot study employing small database, *PloS one* **12**(11), e0187336. doi: 10.1371/journal.pone.0187336.

Chollet, F. (2017). Xception: Deep learning with depthwise separable convolutions, in *Proceedings of the IEEE Conference on Computer Vision and Pattern Recognition*, pp. 1251–1258.

Chu, Z. and Wang, Y. (2012). Incidence of retinopathy of prematurity in mainland of china over the last 20 years, *Zhonghua Yan Ke Za Zhi* **48**(2), 179–183.

Committee for the Classification of Retinopathy of Prematurity (1984). An international classification of retinopathy of prematurity, *Pediatrics* **74**(1), 127–133.

Coscas, G., Cunha-Vaz, J., and Soubrane, G. (2010). Macular edema: Definition and basic concepts, *Macular Edema* **47**, 1–9.

Cover, T. M. and Hart, P. E. (1967). Nearest neighbour pattern classification, *IEEE Transactions in Information Theory* **13**(1), 21–27.

De Fauw, J., Ledsam, J. R., Romera-Paredes, B., Nikolov, S., Tomasev, N., Blackwell, S., Askham, H., Glorot, X., O'Donoghue, B., Visentin, D., *et al.* (2018). Clinically applicable deep learning for diagnosis and referral in retinal disease, *Nature Medicine* **24**(9), 1342–1350.

Decencière, E., Cazuguel, G., Zhang, X., Thibault, G., Klein, J.-C., Meyer, F., Marcotegui, B., Quellec, G., Lamard, M., Danno, R., Elie, D., Massin, P., Viktor, Z., Erginay, A., Laÿ, B., and Chabouis, A. (2013). Teleophta: Machine learning and image processing methods for teleophthalmology, *IRBM* **34**(2), 196–203.

Decencière, E., Zhang, X., Cazuguel, G., Lay, B., Cochener, B., Trone, C., Gain, P., Ordonez, R., Massin, P., Erginay, A., Charton, B., and Klein, J.-C. (2014). Feedback on a publicly distributed image database: The messidor database, *Image Analysis and Stereology* **33**(3), 231–234. doi: 10.5566/ias. 1155, https://www.ias-iss.org/ojs/IAS/article/view/1155.

Deng, J., Dong, W., Socher, R., Li, L. J., Li, K., and Li, F. F. (2009). Imagenet: A large-scale hierarchical image database, in *Proceedings of the IEEE Conference on Computer Vision and Pattern Recognition*, pp. 248–255.

Dietterich, T. G. (2000). Ensemble methods in machine learning, in *International Workshop on Multiple Classifier Systems* (Springer), pp. 1–15.

Drexler, W., Sattmann, H., Hermann, B., Ko, T. H., Stur, M., Unterhuber, A., Scholda, C., Findl, O., Wirtitsch, M., Fujimoto, J. G., *et al.* (2003). Enhanced visualization of macular pathology with the use of ultrahigh-resolution optical coherence tomography, *Archives of Ophthalmology* **121**(5), 695–706.

Dufour, P. A., Ceklic, L., Abdillahi, H., Schroder, S., De Dzanet, S., Wolf-Schnurrbusch, U., and Kowal, J. (2012). Graph-based multi-surface segmentation of oct data using trained hard and soft constraints, *IEEE Transaction on Medical Imaging* **32**(3), 531–543.

Esteva, A., Kuprel, B., Novoa, R. A., Ko, J., Swetter, S. M., Blau, H. M., and Thrun, S. (2017). Dermatologist-level classification of skin cancer with deep neural networks, *Nature* **542**(7639), 115–118.

Falavarjani, K. G., Wang, K., Khadamy, J., and Sadda, S. R. (2016). Ultra-wide-field imaging in diabetic retinopathy; an overview, *Journal of Current Ophthalmology* **28**(2), 57–60.

Farabet, C., Couprie, C., Najman, L., and Lecun, Y. (2012). Learning hierarchical features for scene labeling, *IEEE Transactions on Pattern Analysis and Machine Intelligence* **35**(8), 1915–1929.

Faust, O., Acharya, R., Ng, E. Y.-K., Ng, K.-H., and Suri, J. S. (2012). Algorithms for the automated detection of diabetic retinopathy using digital fundus images: A review, *Journal of Medical Systems* **36**(1), 145–157.

Feichtenhofer, C., Pinz, A., and Zisserman, A. (2016). Convolutional two-stream network fusion for video action recognition, pp. 1933–1941.

Fenner, B. J., Wong, R. L., Lam, W.-C., Tan, G. S., and Cheung, G. C. (2018). Advances in retinal imaging and applications in diabetic retinopathy screening: A review, *Ophthalmology and Therapy* **7**(2), 333–346.

Fong, D. S., Aiello, L., Gardner, T. W., King, G. L., Blankenship, G., Cavallerano, J. D., Ferris, F. L., Klein, R., and Association, A. D. (2004). Diabetic retinopathy, *Diabetes Care* **27**(10), 2540–2553.

Gargeya, R. and Leng, T. (2017). Automated identification of diabetic retinopathy using deep learning, *Ophthalmology* **124**(7), 962–969.

Garvin, M. K., Abramoff, M. D., Wu, X., Russell, S. R., Burns, T. L., and Sonka, M. (2009). Automated 3-d intraretinal layer segmentation of macular spectral-domain optical coherence tomography images, *IEEE Transactions on Medical Imaging* **28**(9), 1436–1447.

Glorot, X., Bordes, A., and Bengio, Y. (2011). Deep sparse rectifier neural networks, in *Proceedings of the 14th International Conference on Artificial Intelligence and Statistics* (JMLR Workshop and Conference Proceedings), pp. 315–323.

Goatman, K. A. (2006). A reference standard for the measurement of macular oedema, *British Journal of Ophthalmology* **90**(9), 1197–1202.

Goh, J. K. H., Cheung, C. Y., Sim, S. S., Tan, P. C., Tan, G. S. W., and Wong, T. Y. (2016). Retinal imaging techniques for diabetic retinopathy screening, *Journal of Diabetes Science and Technology* **10**(2), 282–294.

Good, W. V., for Retinopathy of Prematurity Cooperative Group, E. T., *et al.* (2004). Final results of the early treatment for retinopathy of prematurity (etrop) randomized trial, *Transactions of the American Ophthalmological Society* **102**, 233–250.

Greenspan, H., Van Ginneken, B., and Summers, R. M. (2016). Guest editorial deep learning in medical imaging: Overview and future promise of an exciting new technique, *IEEE Transactions on Medical Imaging* **35**(5), 1153–1159.

Group, E. T. F. R. O. P. C. *et al.* (2003). Revised indications for the treatment of retinopathy of prematurity: results of the early treatment for retinopathy of prematurity randomized trial, *Archives of Ophthalmology* **121**(12), 1684–1696.

Gschließer, A., Stifter, E., Neumayer, T., Moser, E., Papp, A., Pircher, N., Dorner, G., Egger, S., Vukojevic, N., and Oberacher-Velten, I. (2015). Inter-expert and intra-expert agreement on the diagnosis and treatment of retinopathy of prematurity, *American Journal of Ophthalmology* **160**(3), 553–560.

Gulshan, V., Peng, L., Coram, M., Stumpe, M. C., Wu, D., Narayanaswamy, A., Venugopalan, S., Widner, K., Madams, T., Cuadros, J., *et al.* (2016). Development and validation of a deep learning algorithm for detection of diabetic retinopathy in retinal fundus photographs, *Jama* **316**(22), 2402–2410.

Haeker, M., Sonka, M., Kardon, R., Shah, V. A., Wu, X., and Abràmoff, M. D. (2007). Automated segmentation of intraretinal layers from macular optical coherence tomography images, in *Medical Imaging 2007: Image Processing*, Vol. 6512 (SPIE), pp. 385–395.

He, J., Baxter, S. L., Xu, J., Xu, J., Zhou, X., and Zhang, K. (2019). The practical implementation of artificial intelligence technologies in medicine, *Nature Medicine* **25**(1), 30–36.

He, K., Zhang, X., and Ren, S. (2016a). Identity mappings in deep residual networks, in *European Conference on Computer Vision*, pp. 630–645.

He, K., Zhang, X., Ren, S., and Sun, J. (2015a). Delving deep into rectifiers: Surpassing human-level performance on imagenet classification, in *Proceedings of the IEEE International Conference on Computer Vision*, pp. 1026–1034.

He, K., Zhang, X., Ren, S., and Sun, J. (2015b). Spatial pyramid pooling in deep convolutional networks for visual recognition, (IEEE), pp. 1904–1916.

He, K., Zhang, X., Ren, S., and Sun, J. (2016b). Deep residual learning for image recognition, in *Proceedings of the IEEE Conference on Computer Vision and Pattern Recognition*, pp. 770–778.

Hernández-Lobato, D., Martínez-Muóz, G., and Suárez, A. (2013). How large should ensembles of classifiers be? *Pattern Recognition* **46**(5), 1323–1336.

Hinton, G. E. and Salakhutdinov, R. R. (2006). Reducing the dimensionality of data with neural networks, *Science* **313**(5786), 504–507.

Hiroki, M., Tabuchi, H., Nakakura, S., Naofumi, I., Miki, M., and Hiroki, E. (2018). Deep-learning classifier with an ultra-wide-field scanning laser ophthalmoscope detects glaucoma visual field severity, *Journal of Glaucoma* **27**(7), 647–652.

Hoover, A. D., Kouznetsova, V., and Goldbaum, M. (2000). Locating blood vessels in retinal images by piecewise threshold probing of a matched filter response, *IEEE Transactions on Medical Imaging* **19**(3), 203–210, doi: 10.1109/42.845178.

Hu, J., Chen, Y., Zhong, J., Ju, R., and Yi, Z. (2018). Automated analysis for retinopathy of prematurity by deep neural networks, *IEEE Transactions on Medical Imaging* **38**(1), 269–279.

Huang, D., Swanson, E. A., Lin, C. P., Schuman, J. S., Stinson, W. G., Chang, W., Hee, M. R., Flotte, T., Gregory, K., Puliafito, C. A., *et al.* (1991). Optical coherence tomography, *Science* **254**(5035), 1178–1181.

Huang, G., Liu, Z., Van Der Maaten, L., and Weinberger, K. Q. (2017). Densely connected convolutional networks, in *Proceedings of the IEEE Conference on Computer Vision and Pattern Recognition*, pp. 4700–4708.

Huang, G., Sun, Y., Liu, Z., Sedra, D., and Weinberger, K. Q. (2016). Deep networks with stochastic depth, in *European Conference on Computer Vision*, pp. 646–661.

ICROP Committee for Classification of Late Stages ROP (1988). An international classification of retinopathy of prematurity, *Pediatrics* **82**(1), 37–43.

Ioffe, S. and Szegedy, C. (2015). Batch normalization: Accelerating deep network training by reducing internal covariate shift, in *Proceedings of the 32nd International Conference on International Conference on Machine Learning*, Vol. 37, pp. 448–456.

Ju, C., Bibaut, A., and van der Laan, M. (2018). The relative performance of ensemble methods with deep convolutional neural networks for image classification, *Journal of Applied Statistics* **45**(15), 2800–2818.

Kaggle, I. (2016). Diabetic retinopathy detection, *American Academy of Ophthalmology*, 2015. https://www.kaggle.com/c/diabetic-retinopathy-detection.

Kauppi, T., Kalesnykiene, V., Kamarainen, J.-K., Lensu, L., and Sorri, A. R., Iiris (2007). Diaretdb1 diabetic retinopathy database and evaluation protocol, in *Medical Image Understanding and Analysis*, Vol. 2007 (Citeseer), p. 61.

Kauppi, T., Kalesnykiene, V., Kamarainen, J.-K., Lensu, L., Sorri, I., Uusitalo, H., Kälviäinen, H., and Pietilä, J. (2006). Diaretdb0: Evaluation database and methodology for diabetic retinopathy algorithms, *Machine Vision and Pattern Recognition Research Group, Lappeenranta University of Technology, Finland* **73**, 1–17.

Krizhevsky, A., Sutskever, I., and Hinton, G. E. (2012). Imagenet classification with deep convolutional neural networks, *Advances in Neural Information Processing Systems*, 25, 1097–1105.

Lang, A., Carass, A., Swingle, E. K., Al-Louzi, O., Bhargava, P., Saidha, S., Ying, H. S., Calabresi, P. A., and Prince, J. L. (2015). Automatic segmentation of microcystic macular edema in oct, *Biomedical Optics Express* **6**(1), 155 169.

LeCun, Y., Bengio, Y., and Hinton, G. (2015). Deep learning, *Nature* **521**(7553), 436–444.

LeCun, Y., Boser, B. E., Denker, J. S., Henderson, D., Howard, R. E., Hubbard, W. E., and Jackel, L. D. (1990). Handwritten digit recognition with a back-propagation network, *Advances in Neural Information Processing Systems* 2, 396–404.

LeCun, Y., Bottou, L., Bengio, Y., and Haffner, P. (1998). Gradient-based learning applied to document recognition, *Proceedings of the IEEE* **86**(11), 2278–2324.

Li, Z., He, Y., Keel, S., Meng, W., Chang, R. T., and He, M. (2018). Efficacy of a deep learning system for detecting glaucomatous optic neuropathy based on color fundus photographs, *Ophthalmology* **125**(8), 1199–1206.

Li, Z., Guo, C. , Nie, D., Lin, D., Zhu, Y., and Chen, C., Wu, X., Xu, F., Jin, C., Zhang, X., Xiao, H., Zhang, K., Zhao, L., Yan, P., Lai, W., Li, J., Feng, W., Li, Y., Wei Ting, and D.S. Lin, H. (2020). Deep learning for detecting retinal detachment and discerning macular status using ultra-widefield fundus images, *Communications Biology* **3**(1), 1–10.

Lin, D., Xiong, J., Liu, C., Zhao, L., Li, Z., Yu, S., Wu, X., Ge, Z., Hu, X., Wang, B., Fu, M., Zhao, X., Wang, X., Zhu, Y., Chen, C., Li, T., Li, Y., Wei, W., Zhao, M., Li, J., Xu, F., Ding, L., Tan, G., Xiang, Y., Hu, Y., Zhang, P., Han, Y., Li, J.-P. O., Wei, L., Zhu, P., Liu, Y., Chen, W., Ting, D. S. W., Wong, T. Y., Chen, Y., and Lin, H. (2021). Application of comprehensive artificial intelligence retinal expert (care) system: A national real-world evidence study, *The Lancet Digital Health* **3**(8), e486–e495.

Lin, G., Shen, C., Hengel, A. V. D., and Reid, I. (2015). Efficient piecewise training of deep structured models for semantic segmentation, *arXiv preprint arXiv:1504.01013*.

Lin, M., Chen, Q., and Yan, S. (2013). Network in network, *arXiv preprint arXiv:1312.4400*.

Litjens, G., Kooi, T., Bejnordi, B. E., Setio, A. A. A., Ciompi, F., Ghafoorian, M., van der Laak, J. A., Van Ginneken, B., and Sánchez, C. I. (2017). A survey on deep learning in medical image analysis, *Medical Image Analysis* **42**, 60–88.

Long, J., Shelhamer, E., and Darrell, T. (2015). Fully convolutional networks for semantic segmentation, in *Proceedings of the IEEE Conference on Computer Vision and Pattern Recognition*, pp. 3431–3440.

Lynch, S., Shah, A., Folk, J. C., Wu, X., and Abràmoff, M. D. (2017). Catastrophic failure in image-based convolutional neural network algorithms for detecting diabetic retinopathy, *Investigative Ophthalmology & Visual Science* **58**(8), 3776–3776.

Matsuba, S., Tabuchi, H., Ohsugi, H., Enno, H., Ishitobi, N., Masumoto, H., and Kiuchi, Y. (2019). Accuracy of ultra-wide-field fundus ophthalmoscopy-assisted deep learning, a machine-learning technology, for detecting age-related macular degeneration, *International Ophthalmology* **39**(6), 1269–1275.

Ministry of Health of the People's Republic of China (2012), National plan for the prevention and treatment of blindness (2012–2015), *Gazette of the National Health and Family Planning Commission of People's Republic of China*, **8**, 19–22.

Mookiah, M., Acharya, U. R., Martis, R. J., Chua, C. K., Lim, C., Ng, E., and Laude, A. (2013). Evolutionary algorithm based classifier parameter tuning for automatic diabetic retinopathy grading: A hybrid feature extraction approach, *Knowledge-Based Systems* **39**, 9–22. doi: https://doi.org/10.1016/j.knosys.2012.09.008.

Moskowitz, A., Fulton, A. and, Hansen, R. (2016). Retinal, visual, and refractive development in retinopathy of prematurity, *Eye and Brain* **8**(1), 103–111.

Nagasato, D., Tabuchi, H., Ohsugi, H., Masumoto, H., Enno, H., Ishitobi, N., Sonobe, T., Kameoka, M., Niki, M., Hayashi, K., *et al.* (2018). Deep neural network-based method for detecting central retinal vein occlusion using ultrawide-field fundus ophthalmoscopy, *Journal of Ophthalmology* **2018**, 1875431. doi: 10.1155/2018/1875431, https://europepmc.org/articles/PMC6236766.

Nagasato, D., Tabuchi, H., Ohsugi, H., Masumoto, H., Enno, H., Ishitobi, N., Sonobe, T., Kameoka, M., Niki, M., and Mitamura, Y. (2019). Deep-learning classifier with ultrawide-field fundus ophthalmoscopy for detecting branch retinal vein occlusion, *International Journal of Ophthalmology* **12**(1), 94.

Nagiel, A., Lalane, R. A., Sadda, S. R., and Schwartz, S. D. (2016). Ultra-widefield fundus imaging: A review of clinical applications and future trends, *Retina* **36**(4), 660–678.

Niemeijer, M., van Ginneken, B., Russell, S. R., Suttorp-Schulten, M. S., and Abramoff, M. D. (2007). Automated detection and differentiation of drusen, exudates, and cotton-wool spots in digital color fundus photographs for diabetic retinopathy diagnosis, *Investigative Ophthalmology & Visual Science* **48**(5), 2260–2267.

Ning Cheung, T. Y. W. and Paul Mitchell (2010). Diabetic retinopathy, *Lancet* **376**(9735), 124–136.

Ohsugi, H., Tabuchi, H., Enno, H., and Ishitobi, N. (2017). Accuracy of deep learning, a machine-learning technology, using ultra-wide-field fundus ophthalmoscopy for detecting rhegmatogenous retinal detachment, *Scientific Reports* **7**(1), 1–4.

Ophthalmoscopy, D. and Levels, E. (2002). International clinical diabetic retinopathy disease severity scale detailed table.

Papandreou, G., Kokkinos, I., and Savalle, P.-A. (2015). Modeling local and global deformations in deep learning: Epitomic convolution, multiple instance learning, and sliding window detection, in *IEEE Conference on Computer Vision and Pattern Recognition*, pp. 390–399.

Paszke, A., Gross, S., Chintala, S., Chanan, G., Yang, E., DeVito, Z., Lin, Z., Desmaison, A., Antiga, L., and Lerer, A. (2017). Automatic differentiation in pytorch, in *Advances in Neural Information Processing Systems*.

Penha, F. M., Rosenfeld, P. J., Gregori, G., Falcão, M., Yehoshua, Z., Wang, F., and Feuer, W. J. (2012). Quantitative imaging of retinal pigment epithelial detachments using spectral-domain optical coherence tomography, *American Journal of Ophthalmology* **153**(3), 515–523.

Pratt, H., Coenen, F., Broadbent, D. M., Harding, S. P., and Zheng, Y. (2016). Convolutional neural networks for diabetic retinopathy, *Procedia Computer Science* **90**, 200–205.

Qi, X., Zhang, L., Chen, Y., Pi, Y., Chen, Y., Lv, Q., and Yi, Z. (2019). Automated diagnosis of breast ultrasonography images using deep neural networks, *Medical Image Analysis* **52**, 185–198.

Quellec, G., Charrière, K., Boudi, Y., Cochener, B., and Lamard, M. (2017). Deep image mining for diabetic retinopathy screening, *Medical Image Analysis* **39**, 178–193.

Quinn, G. (2005). The international classification of retinopathy of prematurity revisited: An international committee for the classification of retinopathy of prematurity, *Archives of Ophthalmology* **123**(7), 991–999, doi: 10.1001/archopht.123.7.991, https://www.scopus.com/inward/record.uri?eid=2-s2.0-22844447612&doi=10.1001%2farchopht.123.7.991&partnerID=40&md5=97d1bfba73a0b5ca35ac84f2e46024f6, cited By 1928.

Raghavendra, U., Fujita, H., Bhandary, S. V., Gudigar, A., Tan, J. H., and Acharya, U. R. (2018). Deep convolution neural network for accurate diagnosis of glaucoma using digital fundus images, *Information Sciences* **441**, 41–49. doi: https://doi.org/10.1016/j.ins.2018.01.051, https://www.sciencedirect.com/science/article/pii/S0020025518300744.

Resnikoff, S., Felch, W., Gauthier, T.-M., and Spivey, B. (2012). The number of ophthalmologists in practice and training worldwide: a growing gap despite more than 200 000 practitioners, *British Journal of Ophthalmology* **96**(6), 783–787.

Ricard, C. A., Cel, D., and Dammann, O. (2017). Screening tool for early postnatal prediction of retinopathy of prematurity in preterm newborns (step-rop). *Neonatology* **112**(2), 130–136.

Ronneberger, O., Fischer, P., and Brox, T. (2015). U-net: Convolutional networks for biomedical image segmentation, in *International Conference on*

Medical Image Computing and Computer-Assisted Intervention (Springer), pp. 234–241.

Roth, A. M. (1977). Retinal vascular development in premature infants, *American Journal of Ophthalmology* **84**(5), 636–640.

Roy, A. G., Conjeti, S., Karri, S. P. K., Sheet, D., Katouzian, A., Wachinger, C., and Nassir, N. (2017). Relaynet: Retinal layer and fluid segmentation of macular optical coherence tomography using fully convolutional networks, *Biomedical Optics Express* **8**(8), 3627–3642.

Rra, B., Flaxman, S. R., Braithwaite, T., Cicinelli, M. V., Das, A., Jonas, J. B., Keeffe, J., Kempen, J. H., Leasher, J., and Limburg, H. (2017). Magnitude, temporal trends, and projections of the global prevalence of blindness and distance and near vision impairment: A systematic review and meta-analysis, *The Lancet Global Health* **5**(9), e888–e897.

Rubini, S. S. and A. Kunthavai, D. (2015). Diabetic retinopathy detection based on eigenvalues of the hessian matrix, *Procedia Computer Science* **47**, 311–318.

Rumelhart, D. E., Hinton, G. E., and Williams, R. J. (1986). Learning representations by back-propagating errors, *Nature* **323**(6088), 533–536.

Shah, P. K., Prabhu, V., Karandikar, S. S., Ranjan, R., Narendran, V., and Kalpana, N. (2016). Retinopathy of prematurity: Past, present and future, *World Journal of Clinical Pediatrics* **5**(1), 35–46.

Shin, H.-C., Roth, H. R., Gao, M., Lu, L., Xu, Z., Nogues, I., Yao, J., Mollura, D., and Summers, R. M. (2016). Deep convolutional neural networks for computer-aided detection: CNN architectures, dataset characteristics and transfer learning, *IEEE Transactions on Medical Imaging* **35**(5), 1285–1298.

Silva, P. S., Horton, M. B., Clary, D., Lewis, D. G., Sun, J. K., Cavallerano, J. D., and Aiello, L. P. (2016). Identification of diabetic retinopathy and ungradable image rate with ultrawide field imaging in a national teleophthalmology program, *Ophthalmology* **123**(6), 1360–1367.

Silver, D., Huang, A., Maddison, C. J., Guez, A., Sifre, L., Van Den Driessche, G., Schrittwieser, J., Antonoglou, I., Panneershelvam, V., Lanctot, M., *et al.* (2016). Mastering the game of go with deep neural networks and tree search, *Nature* **529**(7587), 484–489.

Simonyan, K. and Zisserman, A. (2014). Very deep convolutional networks for large-scale image recognition, *arXiv preprint arXiv:1409.1556*.

Singh, H., Meyer, A. N., and Thomas, E. J. (2014). The frequency of diagnostic errors in outpatient care: Estimations from three large observational studies involving us adult populations. *BMJ Quality and Safety* **23**(9), 727–731.

Soler, L., Hostettler, A., Agnus, V., Charnoz, A., Fasquel, J., Moreau, J., Osswald, A., Bouhadjar, M., and Marescaux, J. (2010). 3d image reconstruction for comparison of algorithm database: A patient specific anatomical and medical image database, IRCAD, Strasbourg, France, Tech. Rep.

Soliman, A. Z., Silva, P. S., Aiello, L. P., and Sun, J. K. (2012). Ultra-wide field retinal imaging in detection, classification, and management of diabetic retinopathy, in *Seminars in Ophthalmology*, Vol. 27 (Taylor & Francis), pp. 221–227.

Springenberg, J. T., Dosovitskiy, A., Brox, T., and Riedmiller, M. (2014). Striving for simplicity: The all convolutional net, *arXiv preprint arXiv:1412.6806.*

Srivastava, N., Hinton, G., Krizhevsky, A., Sutskever, I., and Salakhutdinov, R. (2014). Dropout: A simple way to prevent neural networks from overfitting, *Journal of Machine Learning Research* **15**(1), 1929–1958.

Staal, J., Abramoff, M. D., Niemeijer, M., Viergever, M. A., and van Ginneken, B. (2004). Ridge-based vessel segmentation in color images of the retina, *IEEE Transactions on Medical Imaging* **23**(4), 501–509, doi: 10.1109/TMI. 2004.825627.

Stark, J. A. (2000). Adaptive image contrast enhancement using generalizations of histogram equalization, *IEEE Transactions on Image Processing* **9**(5), 889–896.

Stark, J. A. and Fitzgerald, W. J. (1994). Model-based adaptive histogram equalization, *Signal Processing* **39**(1-2), 193–200.

Sun, Y., Liang, D., Wang, X., and Tang, X. (2015). Deepid3: Face recognition with very deep neural networks, *arXiv preprint arXiv:1502.00873* .

Szegedy, C., Ioffe, S., Vanhoucke, V., and Alemi, A. (2017). Inception-v4, inception-resnet and the impact of residual connections on learning .

Szegedy, C., Liu, W., Jia, Y., Sermanet, P., Reed, S., Anguelov, D., Erhan, D., Vanhoucke, V., and Rabinovich, A. (2015). Going deeper with convolutions, in *Proceedings of the IEEE Conference on Computer Vision and Pattern Recognition*, pp. 1–9.

Szegedy, C., Vanhoucke, V., Ioffe, S., Shlens, J., and Wojna, Z. (2016). Rethinking the inception architecture for computer vision, in *Proceedings of the IEEE Conference on Computer Vision and Pattern Recognition*, pp. 2818–2826.

Tajbakhsh, N., Shin, J. Y., Gurudu, S. R., Hurst, R. T., Kendall, C. B., Gotway, M. B., and Liang, J. (2016). Convolutional neural networks for medical image analysis: Full training or fine tuning, *IEEE Transactions on Medical Imaging* **35**(5), 1299–1312.

Tamkin, A., Usiri, I., and Fufa, C. (2013). Deep CNNS for diabetic retinopathy detection.

Tasman, W., Patz, A., Mcnamara, J. A., Kaiser, R. S., Trese, M. T., and Smith, B. T. (2006). Retinopathy of prematurity: The life of a lifetime disease, *American Journal of Ophthalmology* **141**(1), 167–174.

Terry, T. L. (1942). Extreme prematurity and fibroblastic overgrowth of persistent vascular sheath behind each crystalline lens from the massachusetts eye and ear infirmary, *American Journal of Ophthalmology* **25**(2), 203–204.

Tieleman, T. and Hinton, G. (2012). Lecture 6.5-rmsprop: Divide the gradient by a running average of its recent magnitude, *COURSERA: Neural Networks for Machine Learning* **4**(2), 26–31.

Ting, D. S. W., Cheung, C. Y.-L., Lim, G., Tan, G. S. W., Quang, N. D., Gan, A., Hamzah, H., Garcia-Franco, R., San Yeo, I. Y., Lee, S. Y., *et al.* (2017). Development and validation of a deep learning system for diabetic retinopathy and related eye diseases using retinal images from multiethnic populations with diabetes, *Jama* **318**(22), 2211–2223.

Ting, K. M. and Witten, I. H. (1999). Issues in stacked generalization, *Journal of Artificial Intelligence Research* **10**, 271–289.

Topol, E. J. (2019). High-performance medicine: The convergence of human and artificial intelligence, *Nature Medicine* **25**(1), 44–56.

Tranos, P. G., Wickremasinghe, S. S., Stangos, N. T., Topouzis, F., Tsinopoulos, I., and Pavesio, C. E. (2004). Macular edema, *Survey of Ophthalmology* **49**(5), 470–490.

Trichonas, G. and Kaiser, P. K. (2014). Optical coherence tomography imaging of macular oedema, *British Journal of Ophthalmology* **98**(Suppl 2), ii24–ii29.

Tsoumakas, G., Partalas, I., and Vlahavas, I. (2008). A taxonomy and short review of ensemble selection, in *Workshop on Supervised and Unsupervised Ensemble Methods and Their Applications*, pp. 1–6.

Udupa, J. K., Leblanc, V. R., Ying, Z., Imielinska, C., Schmidt, H., Currie, L. M., Hirsch, B. E., and Woodburn, J. (2006). A framework for evaluating image segmentation algorithms, *Computerized Medical Imaging and Graphics* **30**(2), 75–87.

Viswanatha, K. *et al.* (2018). Automatic diabetic retinopathy detection using FCM, *Internasional Journal of Engineering Science Invention (IJESI)* **7**(4), 19–24.

Wallace, D. K., Zhao, Z., and Freedman, S. F. (2007). A pilot study using "rop-tool" to quantify plus disease in retinopathy of prematurity, *Journal of American Association for Pediatric Ophthalmology and Strabismus* **11**(4), 381–387.

Walter, T., Klein, J.-C., Massin, P., and Erginay, A. (2002). A contribution of image processing to the diagnosis of diabetic retinopathy-detection of exudates in color fundus images of the human retina, *IEEE Transactions on Medical Imaging* **21**(10), 1236–1243.

Wang, J., Zhang, L., Chen, Y., and Yi, Z. (2017). A new delay connection for long short-term memory networks, *International Journal of Neural Systems* **28**(6), 1750061–1750061.

Wang, S., Yin, Y., Cao, G., Wei, B., Zheng, Y., and Yang, G. (2015). Hierarchical retinal blood vessel segmentation based on feature and ensemble learning, *Neurocomputing* **149** (Part B), 708–717.

Wessel, M. M., Aaker, G. D., Parlitsis, G., Cho, M., D'Amico, D. J., and Kiss, S. (2012). Ultra–wide-field angiography improves the detection and classification of diabetic retinopathy, *Retina* **32**(4), 785–791.

Williams, R. J. and Zipser, D. (1989). A learning algorithm for continually running fully recurrent neural networks, *Neural Computation* **1**(2), 270–280.

Winder, R. J., Morrow, P. J., Mcritchie, I. N., Bailie, J. R., and Hart, P. M. (2009). Algorithms for digital image processing in diabetic retinopathy, *Computerized Medical Imaging and Graphics* **33**(8), 608–622.

Wolf, S. and Wolf-Schnurrbusch, U. (2010). Spectral-domain optical coherence tomography use in macular diseases: A review, *Ophthalmologica* **224**(6), 333–340.

World Health Organization (2013). Universal eye health: a global action plan 2014–2019. https://www.who.int/blindness/actionplan/en/.

World Health Organization (2016). *Global report on diabetes* (World Health Organization).

World Health Organization (2019). World report on vision. https://www.who. int/publicationsdetail/worldreportonvision.

Worrall, D. E., Wilson, C. M., and Brostow, G. J. (2016). Automated retinopathy of prematurity case detection with convolutional neural networks, in *Deep Learning and Data Labeling for Medical Applications*, pp. 68–76.

Xie, L. (2017). Some suggestions on the prevention and treatment of blindness in China, *Chinese Journal of Ophthalmologic Medicine*, **53**(1), 2.

Xu, Y., Yan, K., Kim, J., Wang, X., Li, C., Su, L., Yu, S., Xu, X., and Feng, D. D. (2017). Dual-stage deep learning framework for pigment epithelium detachment segmentation in polypoidal choroidal vasculopathy, *Biomedical Optics Express* **8**(9), 4061–4076.

Yang, Y., Li, T., Li, W., Wu, H., Fan, W., and Zhang, W. (2017). Lesion detection and grading of diabetic retinopathy via two-stages deep convolutional neural networks, in *International Conference on Medical Image Computing and Computer-Assisted Intervention*, Vol. 10435 (Springer, Cham), pp. 533–540.

Yau, G. S., Lee, J. W., Tam, V. T., Yip, S., Cheng, E., Liu, C. C., Chu, B. C., and Wong, I. Y. (2015). Incidence and risk factors for retinopathy of prematurity in multiple gestations: A chinese population study, *Medicine* **94**(18), 185–191.

Yi, Z. (2010). Foundations of implementing the competitive layer model by lotka-volterra recurrent neural networks, *IEEE Transactions on Neural Networks* **21**(3), 494–507.

Yi, Z. and Tan, K. K. (2004). *Convergence Analysis of Recurrent Neural Networks* (Kluwer Academic Publishers, Norwell, MA, USA), ISBN 1402076940.

Zeiler, M. D. (2012). Adadelta: An adaptive learning rate method, *arXiv preprint arXiv:1212.5701*.

Zeiler, M. D. and Fergus, R. (2014). Visualizing and understanding convolutional networks, in D. Fleet, T. Pajdla, B. Schiele, and T. Tuytelaars (eds.), *Computer Vision — ECCV 2014* (Springer International Publishing, Cham), ISBN 978-3-319-10590-1, pp. 818–833.

Zhang, W., Zhong, J., Yang, S., Gao, Z., Hu, J., Chen, Y., and Yi, Z. (2019). Automated identification and grading system of diabetic retinopathy using deep neural networks, *Knowledge-Based Systems* **175**, 12–25.

Zhao, J. *et al.* (2010). Prevalence of vision impairment in older adults in rural china: The china nine-province survey, *Ophthalmology* **117**(3), 409–416.

Zhou, B., Khosla, A., Lapedriza, A., Oliva, A., and Torralba, A. (2016). Learning deep features for discriminative localization, in *2016 IEEE Conference on Computer Vision and Pattern Recognition (CVPR)*, pp. 2921–2929, doi: 10.1109/CVPR.2016.319.

Zhou, Y., Chen, C., Chen, L., *et al.* (2015). Multicenter survey on the clinical features and fundus lesions of retinopathy in premature infants in mainland china, *Chinese Journal of Evidence-Based Pediatrics* **10**, 161–165.

Zuiderveld, K. (1994). Contrast limited adaptive histogram equalization, *Graphics Gems*, pp. 474–485.

Index

A

age-related macular degeneration
  (AMD), 1, 184–185, 187
AI challenger, 140
AlphaGo, 5
annotators, 186–187
artificial intelligence (AI), 3–8
atrous spatial pyramid pooling
  (ASPP), 127–128, 130–131, 134,
  136–138, 140–152, 154–156
augmentation, 69, 72, 75, 79, 97, 142,
  166, 171, 189, 214

B

B/S architecture, 153
backpropagation (BP), 16
binary classification, 189, 193, 196,
  198, 204, 209

C

cataract, 1, 7, 162–163, 187
Chengdu Women and Children's
  Center Hospital, 16, 19, 22, 24, 55,
  60–61
class imbalance, 183, 194, 196, 212
cloud, 153
cloud computing, 11, 17, 63, 71, 86–87
cloud server, 53, 55–56, 153–154
color Doppler, 2, 6

contrast stretching, 97
cross-entropy, 16, 41–42, 105, 142, 170

D

database server, 122
deep convolutional neural network
  (DCNN), 170, 172, 176
deep full connection network
  (DFNN), 170, 172, 176
deep learning (DL), 4–9, 157,
  158–160, 180, 184–185, 212, 213
DeepDR, 89–90, 122, 124–125
DeepLab, 129, 141
DeepLabv, 141–142
DeepOCT, 152–155
DeepROP, 11–12, 17–18, 24–26,
  53–55, 60–61
deeprop, 16
DeepUWF, 157, 159, 180, 214
DeepUWF-Plus, 183–184, 208, 211,
  215
diabetic retinopathy (DR), 1–3, 7–9,
  63–72, 77, 80, 82–84, 86, 89–96,
  99–101, 109, 122, 124–125,
  159–163, 168, 175, 177–180, 184,
  187, 191, 203, 207, 212–213
DIARETDB0, 67–69
DIARETDB0/DIARETDB1, 67
DIARETDB1, 68–69

dice similarity coefficient (DSC), 141,
143–145, 147–148, 150–152, 156
digital retinal images for vessel
extraction (DRIVE), 67–69
DR screening, 91, 99, 115
dropout, 104, 137–139, 170, 194

E

encoder–decoder, 130–131, 155
ensemble, 84, 89, 98, 100–101,
106–107, 109, 113, 120, 122, 167,
173–174, 176, 192, 197, 199–201,
203–206, 208, 212

F

feature aggregate operator, 40–42, 44
feature aggregation, 31
feature extractor, 192–193, 198–201,
207–208
feature map, 15, 39, 42–43, 76, 79, 83
feature-binding, 14–16
fine-tune, 16, 34, 40, 44, 106
five-class, 200
five-class classification, 197, 201, 209,
212
four-class classification, 197, 199–200,
207–208, 210–211
fundus disease screening, 2–3, 6–7,
157, 160, 173, 181
fundus diseases, 1–3, 6–9, 53, 157,
159–161, 166, 176, 179, 187, 198,
215

G

glaucoma, 160–163, 184, 187
grading network (Gr-Net), 11, 14–17,
19, 21–22, 25–26

H

histogram equalization (HE), 96

I

identification network (Id-Net), 11,
14–17, 19, 21–22, 25–26

IDX-DR, 160
inception, 14–16, 31, 34, 40, 42,
44, 77–86, 92, 167, 193, 199,
200
inception-V2, 41–46, 61
InceptionResNetV2, 101, 108–109,
111–112, 172
InceptionV3, 68, 101, 108, 110–112,
114, 116, 117, 123, 167–169, 172,
174–176, 179, 193, 199–200,
204

K

kappa, 168, 171, 174–175, 196, 202,
204, 206

L

learning, 5
limited contrast AHE (CLAHE), 164,
166, 169, 172, 174, 176–179

M

macular edema (ME), 1, 7, 9,
127–130, 132–134, 141, 145,
152–156
minor ROP, 12–13, 19, 21–22, 26
model server, 122
myopia, 157, 159, 161–164, 166, 175,
177, 178–180, 187, 191, 203, 207,
212–213

N

non-proliferative DR (NPDR), 64, 66,
69, 71–72, 90, 95
NPDR2PDR, 94–95, 97, 107

O

ocular fundus disease, 1
one-step classification, 211
one-step strategy, 197, 200–201,
209–210
optical coherence tomography
(OCT), 2, 6, 9, 127–134, 146,
152–155

P

pathological myopia (PM), 1
per-examination, 27, 34, 47
per-image, 34, 45, 47
performance, 143
pigment epithelium detachment
    (PED), 127–129, 131, 140, 143–145,
    147–151, 154, 156
plus, 20, 26–30, 32–34, 57, 61
positive predictive value (PPV),
    143–145, 147, 151–152
preplus, 20, 33
preprocessing, 67, 69, 72, 75, 77, 86,
    96–99, 106, 111, 157, 162, 164, 166,
    171–172, 174, 176–177, 179, 181,
    189
pretraining, 16, 31, 34, 40, 61, 79,
    100, 106, 114, 121, 167, 169, 172,
    180
proliferative DR (PDR), 64, 66,
    71–72, 83, 92, 95, 97, 112

R

rectified linear unit (ReLU), 76
referable diabetic retinopathy (RDR),
    92
RetCam, 27, 29, 35, 51
retinal detachment (RD), 28–29, 37,
    159, 184–185, 187, 188, 191, 200,
    203, 207, 212–213
retinal tear (RT), 187–188, 191, 200,
    203, 207, 212–213
retinopathy of prematurity (ROP), 1,
    7, 11–22, 24–35, 37–40, 43–48,
    50–52, 57, 60–61
RMSprop, 171
ROP grading, 11, 20–21, 25–26
ROP screening, 11–12, 16–20, 24–26
RT&RD, 161, 163, 166, 175, 177–180

S

sensitivity, 11–12, 21, 25
severe ROP, 12–13, 19, 21–22, 26, 32,
    38–39, 44–45, 47

Sichuan Academy of Medical
    Sciences, 92
Sichuan Provincial People's Hospital,
    92, 125
specificity, 11–12, 18, 21, 25
stage, 13, 26–30, 34–35, 37–38, 57,
    61
standard deep neural network
    (SDNN), 89, 101–104, 106, 121
stochastic ASPP (sASPP), 127–128,
    130–131, 134, 137–139, 141–142,
    147–153, 154–156
stochastic gradient descent (SGD),
    171, 194, 197, 199–201
structured analysis of the retina
    (STARE), 67–69
subretinal fluid (SRF), 127–129, 131,
    140, 143–145, 147–150, 154,
    156

T

true positive volume fraction
    (TPVF), 143–145, 147,
    149–151
two-stage, 183, 210, 215
two-step strategy, 208, 210

U

ultrawide-angle fundus, 2, 7, 9
ultrawide-field (UWF), 2, 157–162,
    164, 166–167, 175, 177, 180–181,
    183–187, 193, 211, 215
UWF fundus screening, 159

W

web server, 122, 124
WeChat, 53, 57, 60

X

Xception, 97, 101, 108–109, 111–112,
    116–117, 167–169, 172, 174–176,
    178–179

Z

zone, 13, 26, 28